REVERSING BACK & DISC PAIN: SECRETS TO A PAIN-FREE LIFE

REVERSING BACK & DISC PAIN: SECRETS TO A PAIN-FREE LIFE

DRS. JEREMY & AMELIA RODROCK DC

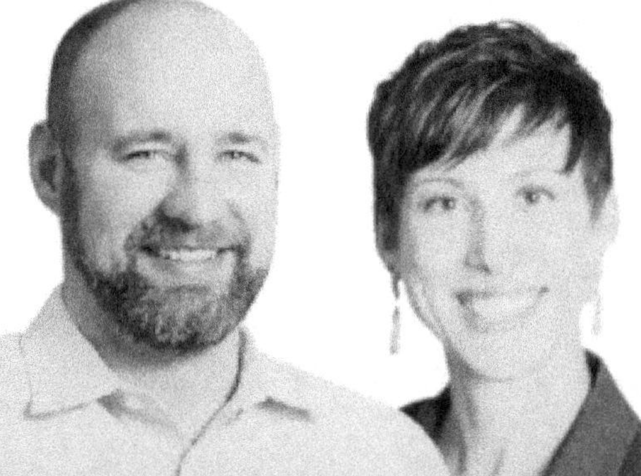

GET ACCESS TO YOUR
FREE REVERSING
SPINE & DISC PAIN
GIFTS BELOW

• Reversing Spine & Disc Pain Guide
• 25 Anti-Inflammatory Recipes
• Free Health Masterclass
• 30-Day Nutrition Plan
• Spine & Disc Pain Relief
  Handbook

RODROCK
CHIROPRACTIC

SCAN ME DR. JEREMY & AMELIA RODROCK, D.C.

CONTENTS

DISCLAIMER

The information provided in this book is intended for educational purposes only and is not a substitute for professional medical advice. The authors and publisher are not liable for any adverse effects or consequences resulting from the use of the information presented herein. Always consult your physician or a qualified healthcare provider regarding any health concerns or before making any decisions related to your health or treatment.

Results may vary based on individual conditions and compliance with the recommended care plan. No guarantees of specific results or outcomes are implied, and painless treatment is not assured. Testimonials reflect individual patient experiences and are not indicative of results for all patients. Fees, discounts, and consultations offered are transparent, and no unrealistic expectations are created. This advertisement complies with the Kansas

State Board of Healing Arts regulations and does not imply superiority over other healthcare providers or methods. Direct solicitation of patients is not employed. For a personalized assessment, please consult with Dr. Jeremy Rodrock, D.C., or Dr. Amelia Rodrock, D.C., licensed in Kansas.

FOREWORD

I still remember the day I met Drs. Jeremy and Amelia Rodrock, D.C.. Their passion for helping people reclaim their lives from the grip of spine and joint pain was palpable. It wasn't just professional dedication; it was a deeply personal mission fueled by a genuine desire to see their patients thrive. As fellow chiropractors and Driven Doc members, we shared a common language, a shared understanding of the intricate ways in which the body can heal, and a shared belief in the power of natural, non-invasive approaches to pain management.

Reading their book, "RESTORE Your Spine," felt like revisiting that first encounter – the passion, the commitment, and the unwavering belief in their patients' potential for healing leaps off every page. But what truly sets this book apart is its practicality. The RESTORE Framework isn't just a theoretical concept; it's a proven, step-by-step program that empowers individuals to take control of their well-being.

This book is a lifeline for anyone struggling with back pain. It debunks common misconceptions, sheds light on the often-overlooked connection between lifestyle choices and spinal health, and provides actionable strategies to manage and even reverse pain naturally. Drs. Jeremy and Amelia don't just offer temporary relief; they guide you towards lasting transformation, empowering you to reclaim your mobility, your energy, and your joy.

If you're tired of living with limitations, if you're searching for a path towards a pain-free life, this book is your guide. Trust in the RESTORE Framework, trust in the expertise of Drs. Jeremy and Amelia Rodrock, and most importantly, trust in your body's incredible capacity for healing. Your journey towards a brighter, more vibrant future starts now.

Dr. Cory Frogley, D.C.

The Data Driven Practice

ABOUT THE AUTHORS

About Dr. Jeremy Rodrock, D.C.

Growing up on a wheat farm in Leoti, Kansas, I learned early on the value of hard work. Those long days instilled in me a deep respect for the land and the satisfaction of a job well done. From a young age, I poured that same energy into every sport imaginable, always pushing my limits and striving for my best. This passion for health and movement led me to pursue a career where I could help others achieve their own optimal well-being.

After graduating from Cleveland Chiropractic College-KC in 2000, I opened my practice in Baldwin City, Kansas, eager to share my knowledge and make a real difference in people's lives. For over two decades, I've had the privilege of helping thousands of patients overcome pain and embrace life to the fullest. Witnessing their transformations fuels my passion every single day.

My amazing wife, Dr. Amelia Rodrock, D.C., is my partner in both life and healing. Together, we're blessed with four incredible children: Myah, Dorreyn, Lillian, and Amelia

Joy. They are my constant reminder of the importance of health and vitality at every stage of life.

My mission as a chiropractor is simple: to empower as many people as possible to live their healthiest, most vibrant lives. It's an honor to share the RESTORE Framework with you in this book, and I truly believe it has the power to transform your life.

Thank you for embarking on this journey with us. Here's to a future filled with joy, movement, and a pain-free spine!

Sincerely,

Dr. Jeremy Rodrock, D.C.

About Dr. Amelia Rodrock, D.C.

My journey into helping the body heal started in my early 20s when I went to massage therapy school. I was fascinated with anatomy and the effect stress had on the muscular system. I was a massage therapist for eight years before I discovered chiropractic. I admit, I did not know anything about chiropractic when I went to chiropractic school. I was a single mother and wanted to provide a better life for my children. And chiropractic seemed the perfect career to do that. And I was right.

After graduating from Cleveland Chiropractic College-KC in 2013, I started my practice in Lawrence, Kansas. Just 20 minutes from my husband's office. I love working with the people in my community and seeing them transform from barely surviving because of pain to thriving and full of life.

As a "middle aged" athlete, I understand the stress we put on our bodies on a daily basis. My passion is to not only help people return to their everyday lives but to help them stay out of pain so they can live life to the fullest every day!

I'm incredibly grateful to share this space with you and hope that the RESTORE Framework empowers you to take control of your spinal health. Here's to a life filled with movement, vitality, and well-being for you and your loved ones!

With heartfelt gratitude,

Dr. Amelia Rodrock, D.C.

1

THE SILENT EPIDEMIC

The phone rang, a frantic voice on the other end. "I threw my back out. I'm in excruciating pain. Can you help?"

It wasn't an unusual call. Back pain, that silent epidemic, touches countless lives, often striking at the most inconvenient times. This time, it was Vanessa, a grandmother visiting from out of town, her weekend plans suddenly derailed by a searing pain in her lower back.

We squeezed her into our schedule, the urgency in her voice mirroring the countless others we'd heard over the years. As she walked in, her face was etched with pain, her movements hesitant, each step a jarring reminder of the invisible enemy that had taken hold.

Skepticism flickered in her eyes as we explained the RESTORE Framework, our holistic approach to pain relief. But as Dr. Jeremy gently adjusted her spine, as she moved through targeted stretches, a gradual shift began to unfold. The tension in her face eased, replaced by a glimmer of hope. Within hours, the excruciating pain that had threatened to steal her weekend had vanished.

"You saved my weekend!" she exclaimed as she left, pain-free and brimming with gratitude. Vanessa's experience is a wonderful example of what's possible with the RESTORE Framework, though it's important to remember that every patient's journey is unique and results can vary.

But for us, it was more than just a saved weekend; it was a powerful reminder of why we do what we do. It was a testament to the transformative potential of the RESTORE Framework, a beacon of hope in the midst of a silent epidemic that has held far too many captive for far too long.

Unmasking the Pain Crisis

A silent epidemic is sweeping the globe. It's not a virus, but its impact is just as real, casting a long shadow over our lives. This epidemic doesn't announce itself with coughs or fevers; it creeps in slowly, a persistent ache in your lower back, a stiffness in your neck that lingers long after you wake. It's the subtle shift in your posture, the way you favor one side, the activities you avoid because they bring a jolt of pain.

You see it everywhere, if you know where to look: in the drawn faces on your morning commute, in the hesitant movements of your aging parents, perhaps even in your own reflection. This is the reality of spine and joint pain, and it's touching countless lives.

But it's time to break the silence. This pervasive suffering thrives in the shadows, dismissed as an inevitable part of aging or a personal weakness. We minimize our experiences, avoid conversations about our discomfort, and accept limitations that we shouldn't have to bear. This isn't about mere physical discomfort; it's about reclaiming agency over our own bodies and lives. It's about seeking solutions, raising awareness, and supporting each other in the quest for lasting relief. This epidemic has held us captive for too long. It's time to fight back.

A Global Burden: The Staggering Reach of Spine and Joint Pain

You are far from alone. The numbers are startling: back pain is the leading cause of disability worldwide, and joint pain affects nearly one in four adults. These statistics represent real people – mothers who can't lift their children, athletes sidelined from their passions, individuals struggling to perform everyday tasks.

This pain knows no boundaries. It transcends age, occupation, and lifestyle. It affects office workers hunched over computers, construction workers bearing heavy loads, and even children burdened by heavy backpacks. The statistics paint a stark picture, but it's the individual stories, the whispers of limitations and lost joys, that reveal the true depth of this crisis.

Beyond the Physical: The Ripple Effect of Chronic Pain

The alarm clock buzzes, but morning brings no real awakening. Just the familiar ache, a unwelcome guest who never leaves. This is the reality of chronic pain – a relentless companion that dictates your every move, a thief robbing you not only of comfort, but of simple joys. It casts a long, persistent shadow that colors every aspect of your day.

Your energy fades, stolen by the constant discomfort. Sleep, once a refuge, becomes elusive. Simple tasks, those things you used to breeze through – picking up your child's scattered toys, laughing with friends over dinner, even drifting off to a peaceful sleep – become monumental hurdles.

And the toll isn't just physical. Relationships strain under the weight of unspoken pain. Anxiety creeps in, a dark whisper that feeds your fears and doubts. Self-doubt blossoms, whispering that you're not enough, that you're letting everyone down. This is the true burden of chronic pain: an isolating, overwhelming weight that affects your mind, body, and spirit.

A Costly Delay: The Price of Ignoring Your Pain

Ignoring your pain won't make it go away – in fact, it often does the opposite. Think of your body like a car: ignoring a small rattle or a flickering engine light might seem harmless at first, but those subtle signs often escalate into costly repairs down the road.

The same principle applies to your spine and joints. What begins as a minor ache, if left unaddressed, can morph into a debilitating condition. That nagging back pain might lead to chronic inflammation, limited mobility, or even disc degeneration. The initial cost of neglecting your well-being is almost always far less than the price you pay later in terms of pain, lost mobility, and diminished quality of life.

Turning Point: The Time for Action is Now

We understand the temptation to downplay pain, to push through discomfort, to hope it will magically disappear. But here's the truth: ignoring the problem won't make it go away. In fact, it often allows it to take root and grow stronger.

You deserve better than a life limited by pain. You deserve to move freely, to embrace life's adventures, and to wake up each morning feeling energized and ready to take on the day. This is about reclaiming your life, not merely managing discomfort. It's about understanding that seeking help isn't a sign of weakness, but a courageous step towards lasting well-being.

Unraveling the Mystery: Getting to the Heart of the Pain Crisis

For far too long, pain has been shrouded in mystery, a frustrating puzzle with seemingly elusive solutions. We're often told to simply "live with it," prescribed medications for temporary relief, or shuffled from one specialist to another without a clear understanding of the root cause. This lack of clarity fuels frustration, delays healing, and perpetuates a cycle of dependence on temporary fixes.

To truly address the pain crisis, we need to shift our perspective. It's time to stop viewing pain as an enemy to be silenced and start seeing it as a messenger, a signal from your body that something needs attention. This journey begins by dispelling the myths that prevent us from finding lasting solutions.

Beyond the Band-Aid: Debunking Common Pain Myths

We often think of pain as a simple alarm system: your finger gets burned, your brain screams "ouch!" But chronic pain is less like a smoke detector and more like a full symphony orchestra playing out of tune. While the initial injury might be the conductor raising the baton, a whole range of instruments chime in to create the experience of pain. We're talking emotions, memories, even our social surroundings – they all add notes to the melody of discomfort.

For years, doctors believed that the severity of an injury directly correlated to the amount of pain experienced. It seemed logical: big injury, big pain, right? Well, now we know it's far more nuanced. Two people with identical injuries can experience completely different pain levels, because individual experiences, past traumas, even cultural expectations shape how our brains interpret pain signals.

This realization is huge. It means that overcoming chronic pain isn't just about treating the physical symptoms – it's about understanding the whole person. True healing requires a holistic approach that addresses the mind and spirit along with the body, like fine-tuning all the instruments for a harmonious performance.

Here are other common misconceptions about pain.

"No pain, no gain" always applies.

While some discomfort is normal during exercise or rehabilitation, persistent pain is your body's way of saying something's wrong. Pushing through significant pain, rather than honoring those signals, can lead to further injury and a longer healing process. It's important to learn the difference between the "good" discomfort of a challenging workout and the sharp, debilitating pain of actual harm.

Pain is just a normal part of getting older.

Many people mistakenly believe that aches, stiffness, and pain are inevitable companions as we age. While it's true that our bodies change over time, significant or persistent pain shouldn't be brushed off as simply a consequence of getting older. Often, underlying conditions, lifestyle factors, or old, untreated injuries are contributing to that pain. Addressing those factors can lead to dramatic improvements, no matter your age.

If the X-ray is clear, the pain must be in my head.

"My X-ray showed nothing, so the doctor said it's probably stress." This all-too-common experience dismisses the very real pain that many people feel, even when imaging doesn't reveal a specific structural issue. X-rays primarily show bones. They often miss soft tissue injuries (like muscle strains, ligament sprains, tendonitis), nerve compression, and other sources of pain. Just because the source of your pain isn't visible on an X-ray doesn't make your experience any less valid or debilitating.

There's a quick fix for chronic pain.

In our instant-gratification world, it's tempting to believe there's a magic pill or one-time treatment that will instantly erase chronic pain. But the reality is that lasting relief requires a more proactive and multi-faceted approach. Think of it like this: chronic pain often develops over time due to a combination of factors - posture problems, repetitive stress, lifestyle choices, even the way we manage stress. Addressing the root cause, not just masking symptoms, takes time, commitment, and a willingness to make lasting changes.

These misconceptions often keep people trapped in a cycle of pain and frustration, preventing them from seeking the help they truly need. It's time to shift the narrative. By understanding that pain, especially chronic pain, is a complex interplay of physical, emotional, and lifestyle factors, we empower ourselves to find lasting solutions that address the root cause, not just the symptoms.

The Lifestyle Link: How Everyday Habits Fuel the Fire

Here's a powerful truth: while genetics and unavoidable injuries play a role, many cases of spine and joint pain are heavily influenced by the choices we make every single day. Our modern lifestyle, for all its conveniences, often sets the stage for pain and dysfunction.

Think of it like this: your body is incredibly resilient, designed to move, adapt, and heal. But when we subject it to repetitive stress, poor posture for hours on end, and a lack of nourishing movement, it's no wonder that pain and stiffness creep in.

Here are a few key lifestyle culprits that often contribute to the epidemic of spine and joint pain:

- **The Sitting Epidemic:** We weren't designed to spend hours upon hours glued to chairs. Prolonged sitting weakens core muscles, tightens hip flexors, and places excessive stress on the discs in your spine. Over time, this can lead to poor posture, back pain, neck pain, and even headaches.
- **The Movement Deficit:** In a world of convenience, we've engineered movement out of our daily lives. We drive instead of walk, take the elevator instead of the stairs, and spend our leisure time scrolling through screens. This lack of natural movement weakens our muscles, reduces flexibility, and increases our risk of injury.
- **Nutrition Neglect:** The old adage "you are what you eat" is especially true when it comes to spine and joint health. A diet high in processed foods, sugar, and unhealthy fats fuels inflammation throughout the body, while a lack of essential nutrients compromises bone density, joint lubrication, and tissue repair.
- **Stress Overload:** Chronic stress does more than just fray our nerves; it wreaks havoc on our physical health as well. When we're constantly stressed, our bodies pump out cortisol, a hormone that, over time, can contribute to inflammation,

muscle tension, and even increased pain perception.

The good news is that recognizing these lifestyle factors empowers you to make different choices. By addressing these often-overlooked contributors to pain, you can create an environment within your body that supports healing, strengthens your spine, and reduces your risk of future injury.

The Silent Saboteur: Inflammation's Role in Chronic Pain

Inflammation: we usually see it as public enemy number one, something to squash with a pill. And while it's true that we don't want inflammation sticking around like an unwelcome house guest, it's important to remember its crucial role in our body's natural healing process.

Think of it as your body's own personal emergency response team. Whether you've tripped and twisted your ankle, sliced a finger while cooking, or feel a nagging ache in your back, your body leaps into action. It dispatches a surge of healing agents to the affected area, increasing blood flow like sirens racing through traffic. These bring in white blood cells – the body's very own clean-up crew – to clear out debris and repair the damage. In these moments, inflammation is our body's best friend, working tirelessly to put us back together.

The trouble begins when this helpful friend outstays its welcome. Chronic inflammation is like that guest who never gets the hint, lingering long after the party's over. This low-level inflammation quietly persists, irritating tissues like an annoying hum you can never quite locate. It contributes to nagging pain, stiffness, and even speeds up the wear and tear on our joints.

The culprits behind chronic inflammation are often the usual suspects: persistent stress, a diet heavy on processed foods, too much time on the couch, and underlying health issues. Fortunately, there's good news! By taking charge of these lifestyle factors and embracing a holistic approach to well-being, we can help our bodies calm the inflammatory storm and break free from the cycle of pain.

Beyond the Physical: The Mind-Body Connection and Its Impact on Pain

We often hear pain described in clinical terms: a pinched nerve, inflammation, muscle strain. But those of us who live with chronic pain know it's so much more than a physical sensation. It seeps into every corner of our lives, a shadow that never quite recedes.

Restless nights bleed into exhausting days. Concentration falters. Simple pleasures, once a source of joy, become frustrating reminders of limitations. Chronic pain doesn't just hurt our bodies; it chips away at our spirit, leaving us grappling with anxiety, isolation, and even despair.

This emotional fallout is not simply a byproduct of pain; it actively fuels the fire. A stressed mind translates to a sensitized nervous system, making us vulnerable to every ache and throb. We find ourselves caught in a vicious cycle where pain intensifies emotional distress, which in turn amplifies the pain itself.

Breaking free requires us to acknowledge this intricate mind-body connection. By treating the emotional and psychological wounds alongside the physical ones, we can begin to soothe the nervous system, dampen the pain signals, and reclaim our lives.

Reaching the Breaking Point: Recognizing When Pain Takes Control

We all experience aches and pains from time to time; it's part of being human. But for millions, pain transforms from a fleeting visitor into an unwelcome houseguest, eventually taking over entire rooms of their lives. It's this transition – from acute, manageable discomfort to chronic, life-altering pain – that marks a critical turning point.

Beyond a Symptom: The Emergence of Pain as a Syndrome

Imagine pain that no longer serves its intended purpose – a helpful alarm system alerting you to injury or illness. Instead, it transforms into a relentless siren, blaring even when there's no immediate threat. This relentless signaling can hijack the nervous system, rewiring its delicate pathways and creating a state of persistent sensitivity.

This is often the point at which pain transcends a mere symptom and evolves into a complex condition known as chronic pain syndrome. This syndrome is characterized by persistent pain that lasts for months or even years, often lingering long after the initial injury has healed.

Chronic pain syndrome is like a tangled web, with physical discomfort intertwined with emotional distress, sleep disturbances, fatigue, and a diminished ability to engage in daily activities. It becomes a vicious cycle: pain leads to anxiety, anxiety amplifies pain perception, sleep suffers, energy plummets, and even the simplest tasks feel overwhelming.

It's crucial to recognize the signs of chronic pain syndrome and understand that reaching this stage is not a sign of weakness. It's a call to action, an opportunity to seek a different approach, one that addresses the multi-faceted nature of this complex condition.

A Slippery Slope: The Allure and Peril of Opioids

We all know that aching, throbbing reminder of an injury or illness – pain. But when it transforms from a fleeting visitor to a constant companion, desperation for relief becomes a way of life. It's no surprise that many turn to the seemingly easiest solution: medication, and specifically, opioids. For years, these potent painkillers were hailed as the miracle cure for those living with moderate to severe pain, offering the hope of reclaimed lives and joyful moments.

Sadly, the reality of opioids often paints a far bleaker picture. Think of it like this – attempting to douse a raging fire by simply tossing a blanket on top. Sure, you might momentarily conceal the flames, but the fire rages on beneath the surface, eventually breaking through with renewed fury. Similarly, while opioids might offer a fleeting reprieve from pain's clutches, they do little to address its root cause. The underlying issues persist, and in many cases, worsen over time, leaving individuals trapped in a cycle of dependence and despair.

Beyond their limited effectiveness in addressing chronic pain, opioids come with a host of serious risks, including:

- **Tolerance and Dependence:** Over time, your body can become accustomed to the effects of opioids, requiring higher and higher doses to achieve the same level of pain relief. This often leads to dependence, both physical and psychological, making it incredibly difficult to stop taking these medications even if you want to.

- **Addiction:** The line between dependence and addiction can be blurry. When the use of opioids becomes compulsive, driven by cravings and a desperate need to avoid withdrawal symptoms, addiction has taken hold, often with devastating consequences for individuals and families.

- **Side Effects:** Opioids come with a laundry list of potential side effects, including drowsiness, constipation, nausea, slowed breathing, and impaired cognitive function. These side effects can significantly impact your quality of life and even lead to other health complications.

The opioid crisis has gripped our nation, highlighting the urgent need for safer, more effective alternatives to chronic pain management. It's time to move beyond the quick-fix mentality and embrace solutions that address the root cause, not just the symptoms, of pain.

A Life Half Lived: The Insidious Erosion of Quality of Life

Chronic pain is a thief. It doesn't just steal your physical comfort, it robs you of the simple joys that make life worth living. What was once effortless – chasing your kids in the park, laughing with friends over dinner, losing yourself in a beloved hobby – can become a distant, painful echo.

The everyday things others take for granted? They transform into Herculean tasks. Getting dressed becomes a marathon. Stairs feel like mountains. Sleep, that precious respite, turns into a nightly battle. This relentless struggle to simply exist can trap you in a cage of isolation. The world shrinks as you decline invitations, avoid cherished activities, and grapple with the fear of becoming a burden to those you love.

Chronic pain whispers insidious doubts, chipping away at your spirit. Energy dwindles, sleep becomes elusive, and focus wavers like a candle in the wind. It's hard to engage, hard to connect, hard to simply be in the present moment when your body feels like a constant source of betrayal. This slow erosion of your life can leave you feeling lost, alone, adrift in a body that feels more like a prison than a home.

Taking Back Control: The Empowering Decision to Seek Help

Hitting rock bottom with chronic pain is awful. You feel robbed, depleted - like pain has squeezed all the joy out of life. But you know what? Sometimes, that awful feeling becomes a turning point.

Because when the pain gets so bad you can't ignore it any longer, you're finally ready for a change. This isn't about some miracle cure; it's about deciding you deserve better. It's about taking charge of your well-being and seeking help, not as a surrender, but as a powerful act of self-care.

That's where we come in. At Rodrock Chiropractic, we get how deeply spine and joint pain affects you. We don't offer band-aid solutions – we work with you to find the source of your pain and build a personalized plan for lasting relief. We believe in empowering you to regain control of your health and your life.

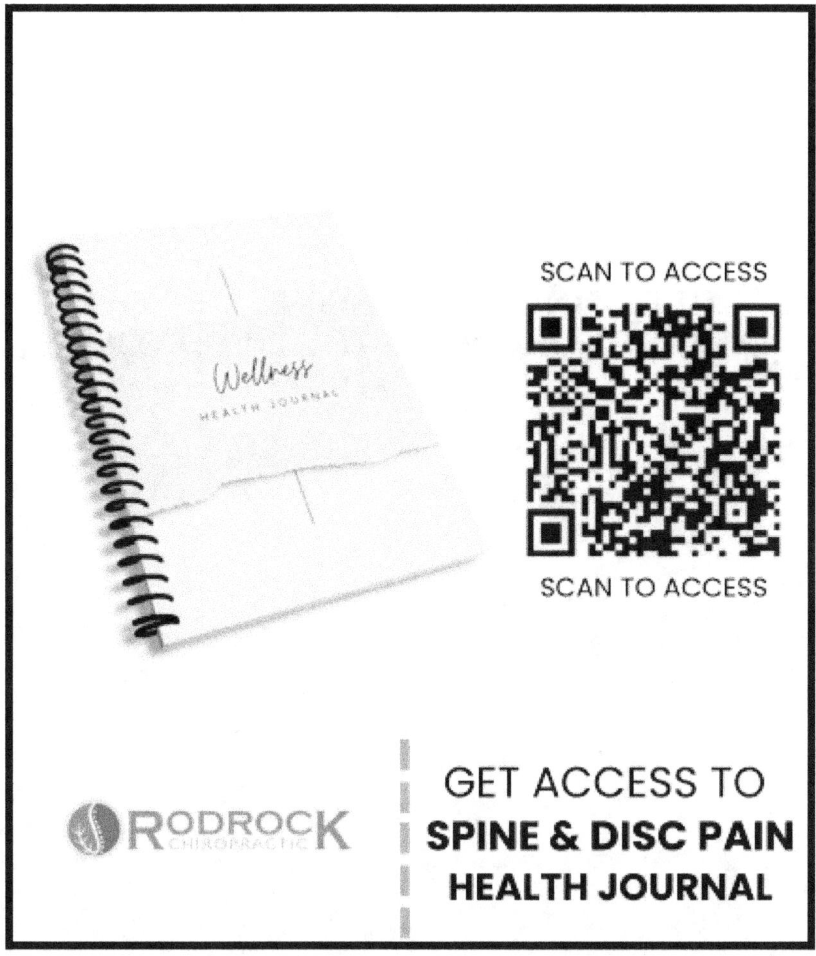

Don't let pain hold you back another day. Call 785-465-5605 and start your journey toward pain relief now.

** Individual results may vary. Please review the disclaimer after the Table of Contents.*

EMBRACING A NEW HORIZON: HOPE AND HEALING WITH THE R.E.S.T.O.R.E. FRAMEWORK

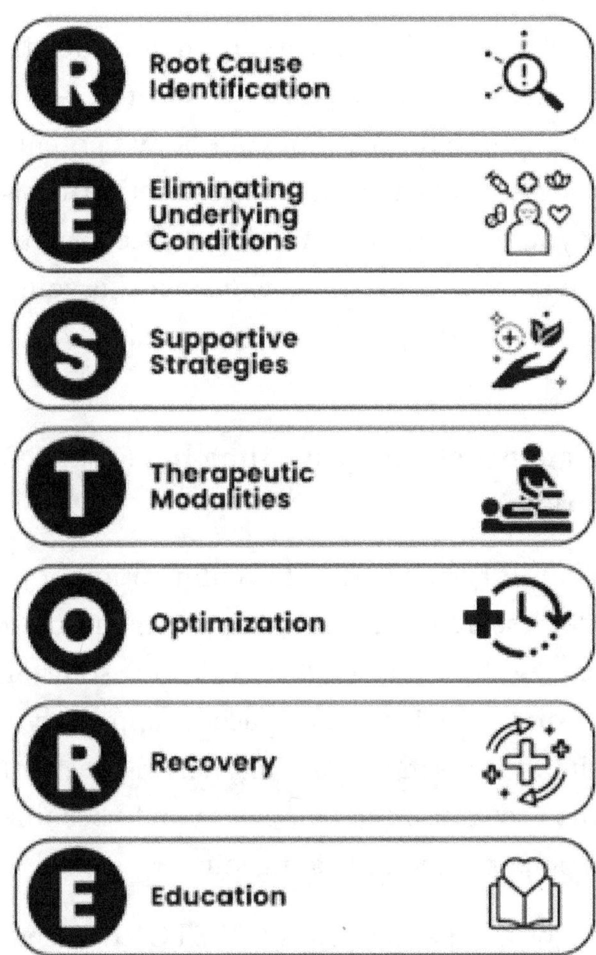

Tired of your back or joint pain dictating your life? You're not alone. Countless remedies promise the world, yet deliver mere whispers of relief. But what if true freedom from pain wasn't a fantasy, but a tangible possibility waiting to be unlocked?

Enter the RESTORE Framework. It's not a quick fix – it's a revolution. This approach goes beyond surface-level treatments, delving into the heart of your body's potential to heal. It's a personalized journey of restoration, designed to empower you to move, live, and thrive, free from the shackles of chronic discomfort. Consider this your invitation to rediscover the joy of living, unburdened.

A Roadmap to Wellness: Unveiling the R.E.S.T.O.R.E. Framework

The RESTORE Framework is the culmination of years of experience, research, and a deep commitment to providing our patients with the most effective, lasting solutions for spine and joint pain. It's a multi-faceted approach that goes beyond simply masking symptoms, delving deeper to address the root cause and empower you to become an active participant in your healing journey.

Let's break down the elements of RESTORE, each letter representing a critical step towards lasting relief and optimal well-being:

R – Root Cause Identification: Instead of chasing symptoms, we start by conducting a thorough assessment to uncover the underlying factors contributing to your pain. This involves listening intently to your story, understanding your health history, and performing comprehensive exams to identify postural imbalances, movement restrictions, and potential areas of dysfunction.

E – Eliminating Underlying Conditions: Once we've identified the root cause, we develop a personalized plan to address any underlying conditions that may be contributing to your pain. This might include addressing nutritional deficiencies, optimizing gut health, correcting postural imbalances, or resolving muscle imbalances.

S – Supportive Strategies: True healing is a partnership. We empower you with the knowledge, tools, and strategies you need to actively participate in your recovery and make sustainable lifestyle changes. This might include personalized exercise plans, ergonomic assessments, stress reduction techniques, or nutritional guidance.

T – Therapeutic Modalities: We utilize a variety of gentle, effective therapies to reduce pain, restore proper joint mechanics, and promote healing. These may include chiropractic adjustments, soft tissue therapies, acupuncture, decompression therapy, and other evidence-based modalities tailored to your unique needs.

O – Optimization: Our focus extends beyond pain relief to encompass whole-person wellness. We help you optimize your overall health and well-being through tailored lifestyle recommendations, nutritional counseling, stress management techniques, and strategies for improving sleep and energy levels.

R – Recovery: We provide ongoing support and guidance throughout your healing journey, adjusting your care plan as needed and celebrating your progress along the way. Our goal is to empower you with the knowledge and tools you need to manage your pain effectively and prevent future recurrences.

E – Education: Knowledge is power. We believe that informed patients are empowered patients. We take the time to educate you about your condition, the mechanics of your body, and the rationale behind our approach, so you can make informed decisions about your health.

Awakening Your Inner Healer: The Power of Your Body's Innate Intelligence

Our bodies are symphonies of resilience, each beat of our hearts a testament to their tireless pursuit of equilibrium. The RESTORE Framework recognizes this intricate dance of self-healing and self-regulation, acknowledging that true healing blossoms from within, not from external interventions seeking a fleeting resolution.

Visualize your body as a tranquil garden, governed by an ancient wisdom that nurtures growth and harmony. Pain or illness resemble encroaching weeds, their presence indicating that this innate wisdom faces obstacles in its pursuit of balance.

The RESTORE Framework seeks to gently uproot these obstacles, empowering your body's innate healing mechanisms to flourish once more. This is not a hostile takeover but a collaboration, a tender cultivation of the body's inherent capacity for restoration, allowing balance to be reclaimed, pain to subside, and optimal health to blossom anew.

A Symphony of Healing: Why the RESTORE Framework Delivers Results

What sets the RESTORE Framework apart is its comprehensive and individualized approach. Rather than relying on a single modality or addressing only the symptoms, we look at the whole person, taking into account the interconnectedness of your physical, emotional, and lifestyle factors.

Our holistic approach combines the best of evidence-based practices, including:

- **Chiropractic Care:** Gentle, precise adjustments to the spine help to restore proper joint alignment, reduce nerve interference, and improve overall nervous system function.

- **Acupuncture:** This ancient practice utilizes strategically placed, ultra-thin needles to stimulate specific points along the body's energy meridians, promoting pain relief, reducing inflammation, and restoring balance.
- **Cutting-Edge Technology:** We incorporate the latest advancements in pain management, such as SoftWave therapy, spinal decompression, and Red Light therapy to accelerate healing and enhance the effectiveness of our treatments.

By combining these modalities in a personalized treatment plan, we create a synergistic effect that addresses your unique needs and goals, leading to more effective and lasting relief.

Embarking on Your Healing Journey: What to Expect on the Path Ahead

We understand that beginning a new approach to pain management can feel both exciting and daunting. That's why we're committed to guiding you every step of the way, providing support, education, and encouragement throughout your journey with us.

In the chapters that follow, we'll delve deeper into each element of the RESTORE Framework, providing practical tools, evidence-based strategies, and inspiring success stories to empower you to take control of your health and reclaim a life free from limitations. We'll explore the profound impact of lifestyle choices, from the foods you eat and the way you move to the thoughts you think and the connections you cultivate.

A Deeper Dive: Looking Beyond the Symptoms to Find Lasting Relief

We've all been there – a leaky faucet, driving you mad with its relentless *drip, drip, drip*. You could grab a bucket, but that's just ignoring the real issue, right? You need to get to the source of the leak, fix that pipe, and silence that incessant dripping for good.

The problem is, most pain management strategies treat your pain like that bucket – they mask the symptoms with medication or quick fixes, offering temporary relief. But they often fall short of addressing the root cause, trapping you in a cycle of discomfort and dependency.

That's where the RESTORE Framework diverges. We believe in finding the leaky pipe in your pain – uncovering the root cause and addressing it head-on. Only then can you truly escape the cycle and embrace lasting relief.

Connecting the Dots: The Power of a Holistic Perspective

The human body isn't a jigsaw puzzle of independent pieces, but a symphony of interconnected systems, each playing a vital role in the grand performance of life. It's within this understanding that we approach pain relief - not with tunnel vision, but with a wide-angle lens that captures the entire panorama of your well-being.

That persistent ache in your lower back might be whispering a tale of muscular imbalances, perhaps tight hamstrings pulling on your pelvis. Or it could be a signal from your constantly engaged stress response system, a reminder that mental tension can manifest physically. And that relentless headache? It might stem from poor posture at your workstation or an unnoticed sensitivity to certain foods.

By acknowledging this intricate dance between body, mind, and spirit, by embracing the interconnectedness within, we can finally design a personalized roadmap to recovery. It's about addressing the root cause of your pain, peeling back the layers to reveal the source of discomfort, and ultimately empowering you to reclaim control of your well-being.

Shifting the Paradigm: From Quick Fixes to Sustainable Healing

True healing isn't a finish line you cross, but a winding path you choose to walk. It's about continually discovering yourself, stepping into your power, and making decisions that fuel your body's remarkable ability to mend. The

RESTORE Framework acts like a trusty compass and toolkit on this journey, providing you with the knowledge, techniques, and strategies to become the architect of your own recovery and cultivate enduring change.

This journey requires abandoning the allure of instant solutions. It's about embracing the reality that profound healing unfolds over time, requiring patience, dedication, and an openness to integrating new habits. Instead of simply silencing the body's cries for help, it's about delving deeper to understand their origin. It's about handing you the reins, enabling you to cultivate lasting lifestyle changes that nurture your overall health and well-being.

Sustainable healing necessitates a profound shift in perspective—a transformation from passive patient to a passionate advocate for your own body. It's about learning to listen to its whispers and roars, deciphering its unique language, and making choices that respect its innate wisdom.

Knowledge is Power: Embracing Education as a Cornerstone of Healing

We believe that informed patients are empowered patients. That's why education is a cornerstone of the RESTORE Framework. We take the time to explain your condition clearly, demystify complex medical jargon, and answer your questions thoroughly.

We want you to understand not just *what* we're doing, but *why* we're doing it. We'll teach you about the mechanics of your body, the factors that contribute to pain, and the science behind our approach. This empowers you to make informed decisions about your health, to actively participate in your healing journey, and to become the best possible advocate for your own well-being.

Your Path to Wellness: The RESTORE Promise

Embarking on any healing journey requires a leap of faith – a belief that something better is possible, a willingness to embrace change, and a commitment to partnering with practitioners who share your vision for optimal well-being.

The RESTORE Framework is more than just a treatment plan; it's a promise – a commitment to providing you with the highest quality care, unwavering support, and the knowledge you need to reclaim your health and live a life free from limitations.

Setting the Stage for Success: What to Expect on Your RESTORE Journey

We believe in transparency and open communication. From the moment you walk through our doors, you can expect:

- **A Warm, Welcoming Environment:** Our team is dedicated to creating a safe, supportive space where you feel heard, respected, and empowered. We believe that healing thrives in an atmosphere of compassion, collaboration, and genuine care.

- **Thorough, Individualized Assessments:** We don't believe in cookie-cutter solutions. We'll take the time to understand your unique story, health history, and goals. We'll conduct comprehensive exams to identify the root cause of your pain and develop a personalized treatment plan tailored to your specific needs.

- **Clear Explanations and Empowering Education:** We'll explain your condition in a way that makes sense, demystify complex medical jargon, and answer your questions thoroughly. We believe that knowledge is power and that informed patients are best equipped to make decisions about their health.

- **A Collaborative Approach:** We believe that true healing is a partnership. We'll work collaboratively with you, respecting your preferences, and involving you in every step of the decision-making process.

- **Gentle, Effective Therapies:** Our approach combines the best of traditional wisdom and cutting-edge technology, always with your safety and comfort in mind.

- **Ongoing Support and Guidance:** We're here for you every step of the way, providing encouragement, adjusting your care plan as needed, and celebrating your progress.

The RESTORE Framework is a roadmap to lasting relief and a life lived on your own terms.

A Journey, Not a Destination: Navigating the Path to Recovery

Healing is less like a straight line, and more like a winding path through nature. Some days you'll breeze along, sunlight dappling the trail ahead. Other days might find you navigating rocky patches, unsure of your footing. Both experiences are part of the journey. The RESTORE Framework doesn't ask for flawlessness, but for acceptance of this very real process. It encourages you to celebrate each small victory, to find joy in those moments where the path feels clear, and to trust the remarkable capacity of your body to mend and recover.

Consider us your partners on this journey. We'll be right there alongside you, offering encouragement, our knowledge in this field, and tailoring your care plan to adapt to your individual needs and progress. We're dedicated to providing you with the resources and support to help ease your discomfort, navigate challenges, and stay motivated as you move toward a healthier, more vibrant you.

Breaking Free: Releasing the Grip of Dependence

Living with chronic pain can feel like being trapped in a revolving door of temporary fixes. You rely on painkillers, muscle relaxants, injections…anything to silence the symphony of aches in your body. But these solutions are fleeting, like band-aids on a gaping wound. Each pill, each treatment, might offer a brief respite, but the cycle always repeats, leaving you caught in a web of dependency and diminishing returns.

This is where the RESTORE Framework comes in. Instead of masking the pain, it helps you understand its origin story, providing you with the tools and knowledge to rewrite your own narrative. Through targeted self-care strategies and by harnessing your body's incredible capacity for healing, the framework guides you toward lasting relief and empowers you to reclaim authority over your health.

Investing in Your Future: A Lifetime of Health and Vitality

Our vision for you extends far beyond pain relief; we want you to experience the joy of true well-being – a life filled with vitality, movement, and the freedom to pursue your passions without limitations.

The RESTORE Framework provides a solid foundation for a lifetime of health. As you progress through your jour-ney, you'll gain valuable knowledge, practical skills, and a deep understanding of your body's needs. These tools will empower you to make choices that support your long-term health, prevent future pain and injury, and embrace life with renewed energy and enthusiasm.

This is about more than just fixing a problem; it's about unlocking a world of possibilities. Are you ready to begin?

Contact us today to schedule an appointment and embark on your journey toward lasting relief and a lifetime of vibrant health. Visit our website or contact our Lawrence or Baldwin City locations at 785-465-5605. Please be advised that scheduling an appointment or undergoing treatment does not guarantee specific results. Individual health outcomes can vary.

Real Patients, Real Results

Grant's Back Pain Breakthrough: Relief in Just One Visit

"I have been fighting lower back and mid back pain for about a month. I got scheduled in no time, and after the first visit, I felt so much better! Great and friendly staff! Highly recommend!"

Cindy's 5-Star Review: Dr. Rodrock's Kind & Professional Care

"I've had major challenges with my back all of my life. I've always chosen chiropractic care as my method for pain management. I've never had such great results as I have since going to Dr. Rodrock. The office staff being incredibly kind is a nice bonus as well. I'm very pleased with the all-around professionalism and KINDNESS. 5 stars and then some!"

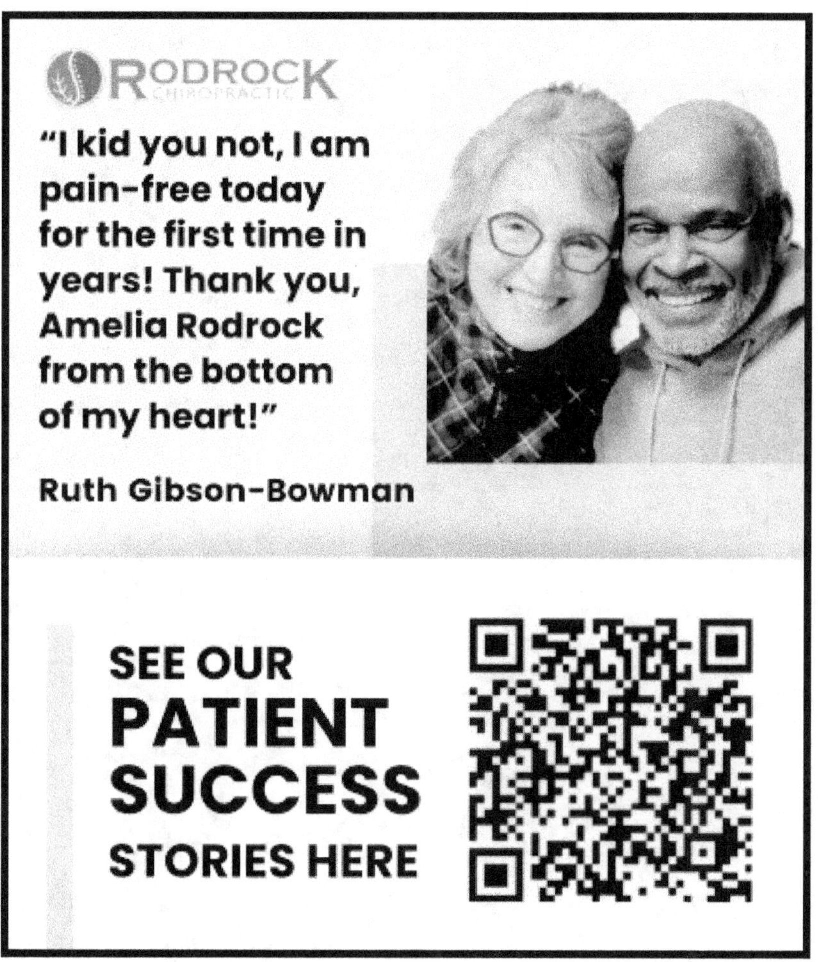

* These testimonials reflect individual experiences and results,

which may vary. They are not intended to represent or guarantee that everyone will achieve the same or similar outcomes.

Ready for lasting relief? Call 785-465-5605 today and discover how to reverse your back and neck pain for good.

** Individual results may vary. Please review the disclaimer after the Table of Contents.*

3

BEYOND THE QUICK FIX: WHY LASTING RELIEF REQUIRES A DIFFERENT APPROACH

Why Quick Fixes Often Fail in the Long Run

Pain relief is a universal desire, and the temptation to opt for quick fixes is undeniable. However, seeking solely to eliminate pain without addressing its root cause can lead to ineffective treatments and potential complications. Just as a bandage cannot mend a broken bone, short-term solutions often fail to provide comprehensive healing for spine and joint pain.

This chapter critically analyzes common quick-fix approaches, shedding light on their inherent limitations, potential risks, and the reasons behind their often temporary results. Our aim is to empower you with knowledge to make informed decisions about your musculoskeletal health. By understanding the complexities of pain management, you can pursue treatments that offer genuine and sustainable healing rather than mere symptom suppression.

The Allure and Illusion: Unmasking the Painkiller Trap

When faced with pain, reaching for a painkiller seems like the most natural response. Over-the-counter or prescription NSAIDs (nonsteroidal anti-inflammatory drugs) and opioids can indeed help alleviate discomfort by reducing inflammation and blocking pain signals. But it's crucial to remember that they only address the symptom, not the root cause of your discomfort.

Think of it like this: covering a fire with a blanket might temporarily conceal the flames and reduce the heat, but the fire is still burning beneath the surface. Similarly, painkillers might provide temporary relief, but the underlying issue persists.

Furthermore, long-term reliance on these medications can have severe consequences. Stomach ulcers, liver damage, kidney problems, and an increased risk of heart attack and stroke are all potential side effects. It's also important to be aware of the potential for dependence or addiction, especially when it comes to opioids.

Weighing the Risks: When Invasive Procedures Fall Short

Invasive procedures, such as spinal injections or surgery, are often presented as last-resort options for spine and joint pain. While these procedures can provide relief in certain cases, they come with inherent risks, lengthy recovery periods, and no guarantee of long-term success.

Spinal injections, for example, often involve injecting corticosteroids (powerful anti-inflammatories) into the epidural space of the spine, aiming to reduce inflammation and alleviate pain. While these injections can provide temporary relief for some individuals, the effects are often short-lived, and repeated injections can weaken surrounding tissues and increase the risk of complications.

Surgery, the most invasive option, is typically reserved for severe cases that haven't responded to more conservative treatments. Spinal surgery is a major procedure with significant risks, including infection, nerve damage, chronic pain, and a lengthy and often challenging rehabilitation process. It's crucial to remember that surgery doesn't address the underlying lifestyle, postural, or biomechanical factors that might have contributed to the problem in the first place, meaning the pain can often return even after a seemingly successful procedure.

Beyond the Band-Aid: Addressing the Limitations of Conventional Approaches

Conventional medicine has made remarkable strides in treating acute injuries and life-threatening diseases. However, when it comes to chronic pain, particularly spine and joint pain, the conventional model often falls short. This is largely because it tends to focus on symptom suppression rather than root cause resolution.

Imagine taking your car to a mechanic because the engine is making a strange noise. Would you be satisfied if the mechanic simply covered the engine with sound-dampening material, masking the noise but leaving the underlying problem unaddressed? Of course not! Yet, this is often how pain is treated within the conventional model – silencing the body's alarm signals without addressing the underlying malfunction.

This approach often leads to a revolving door of treatments, leaving patients feeling frustrated, unheard, and dependent on medications or procedures that provide temporary relief at best.

The Power of Belief: Recognizing the Placebo Effect and False Hope

We humans are capable of remarkable things, and the placebo effect stands as a testament to the sheer power of our minds. This curious phenomenon, where a person benefits from treatment with no real medical value – a sugar pill or a pretend procedure – underscores the intricate dance between our minds and bodies, revealing our innate capacity for healing.

However, this same power can be misleading, especially when it comes to something as debilitating as chronic pain. The allure of a quick fix is undeniable, and many heavily marketed "miracle cures" capitalize on this, their promises echoing with the seductive whisper of the placebo effect. Temporary relief might appear, but like a desert mirage, it soon fades, leaving behind a trail of wasted time, money, and hope.

Therefore, skepticism should be our closest ally when navigating the labyrinth of treatment claims. Look beyond the glossy brochures and dramatic testimonials. Delve into the science, seek evidence-based approaches, and rely on reputable sources. Remember, true healing is a journey, not a race. It's a process demanding patience, dedication, and a commitment to nurturing the whole self.

Separating Fact from Fiction: Why Trendy Approaches Often Fall Short

In the world of health and wellness, there's no shortage of enticing promises – miracle cures, rapid weight loss solutions, and of course, quick fixes for chronic pain. While these fads might offer a glimmer of hope, they often fade as quickly as they appear, leaving a trail of disillusioned individuals and empty wallets in their wake.

This section explores why these trendy approaches often fail to deliver on their lofty promises, particularly when it comes to spine and joint health. Our goal is to empower you with the knowledge to navigate this overwhelming landscape, make informed decisions, and invest in solutions that stand the test of time.

The Allure (and Illusion) of Trendy Diets and Supplements

When it comes to pain relief, fad diets and supplements often take center stage, promising to reduce inflammation, rebuild cartilage, and magically erase discomfort. While some dietary changes and targeted supplementation *can* support overall health and potentially ease certain types of pain, it's essential to approach these trends with a discerning eye.

Here's why many trendy diets and supplements fall short:

- **Oversimplification:** Pain, especially chronic pain, is rarely caused by a single dietary factor. While eliminating certain foods or adopting a restrictive diet might provide temporary relief for some individuals, it rarely addresses the multifaceted nature of chronic pain.
- **Lack of Scientific Rigor:** Many trendy diets and supplements lack robust scientific evidence to support their claims. Testimonials and anecdotal evidence might be compelling, but they shouldn't be mistaken for rigorous scientific proof.
- **The Band-Aid Effect:** Even if a particular diet or supplement provides temporary relief, the benefits often fade once you stop following the restrictive

protocol. True healing requires sustainable lifestyle changes, not quick fixes.

- **Potential for Harm:** Some restrictive diets can lead to nutrient deficiencies, while certain supplements might interact negatively with medications or have unintended side effects. It's always best to consult with a qualified healthcare professional before making significant changes to your diet or supplement regimen.

Beware of False Promises: The Problem with "Miracle" Cures

The term "miracle cure" itself should raise a red flag. Chronic pain, particularly when it involves the intricate structures of the spine and joints, is rarely resolved with a single treatment or product, no matter how enticing the marketing claims.

The problem with miracle cures often lies in their:

- **Overblown Claims:** Miracle cures often prey on desperation, promising unrealistic results and timelines. They might use testimonials, before-and-after photos, or anecdotal evidence to support their claims, but these lack the rigor of scientific studies.
- **Ignoring the Complexity of Pain:** Chronic pain is often multifaceted, involving a complex interplay

of physical, emotional, and lifestyle factors. Miracle cures tend to oversimplify the problem, suggesting that a single product or treatment can address all these interconnected elements.

- **Distracting from Sustainable Solutions:** The allure of a quick fix can distract individuals from pursuing evidence-based approaches that require more time, effort, and commitment but ultimately offer more sustainable results.

Beyond the Hype: The Truth About Detoxes and Cleanses

Detox teas, juice fasts, colonics – the world of detoxification is rife with promises to purify your body, eliminate toxins, and even alleviate pain. While it's true that we live in a world saturated with environmental toxins and that supporting your body's natural detoxification processes is essential for overall health, the claims surrounding these trendy cleanses often lack scientific support.

Here's the reality:

- **Your Body is a Self-Cleaning Machine:** Your liver, kidneys, digestive system, and lymphatic system work tirelessly to filter toxins and eliminate waste. While supporting these organs through a nutrient-rich diet, adequate hydration, and stress management is important, drastic detox protocols are rarely necessary.

- **More Hype than Substance:** Many detox products and cleanses lack scientific evidence to back up their claims. In fact, some can even be harmful, leading to dehydration, electrolyte imbalances, or digestive upset.
- **Sustainability Over Quick Fixes:** True detoxification is about adopting long-term healthy habits, not punishing your body with short-term restrictions.

Finding Clarity Amidst the Chaos: Navigating the World of Pain Relief Options

In today's information age, we're bombarded with health advice from every direction – social media influencers touting the latest supplements, celebrity doctors promoting trendy treatments, and countless websites promising quick fixes for every ailment. It can feel over-whelming, even paralyzing, to sift through this constant barrage of information and discern fact from fiction.

So how do you cut through the noise and make informed decisions about your spine and joint health? Here are some key strategies:

- **Consult with Qualified Healthcare Professionals:** Seek guidance from licensed healthcare providers who focus on musculoskeletal health, such as chiropractors, physical therapists, or orthopedic doctors. These professionals can provide personalized evaluations, recommend treatments backed by scientific research, and help you understand the various options available for managing your discomfort.

- **Prioritize Evidence over Hype:** Look for treatments and therapies backed by scientific research, not just anecdotal evidence or marketing hype. Reputable practitioners will be transparent about the evidence supporting their methods and be willing to answer your questions thoroughly.

- **Tune into Your Body's Signals:** Your body is incredibly intelligent and constantly communicates its needs. Pay attention to how your body responds to different treatments, foods, movements, and lifestyle changes. What works for one person might not work for another, so listen to your own internal wisdom and advocate for your individual needs.

- **Embrace a Holistic Perspective:** True healing rarely comes from a single solution. Explore approaches that address the interconnectedness of your physical, emotional, and lifestyle factors.

- **Be Patient and Persistent:** Healing is a journey, not a destination. It takes time, commitment, and a willingness to experiment and adjust your approach along the way. Don't be discouraged if you encounter setbacks or plateaus. Every step you take towards understanding your body and making choices that support its natural healing abilities is a step in the right direction.

The allure of a quick fix for pain is powerful, especially when it comes wrapped in trendy packaging or promises of miraculous results. But true, lasting healing requires a more discerning approach—one grounded in evidence, personalized care, and a deep understanding of your body's innate healing wisdom. Don't be swayed by the latest fads or seduced by unrealistic promises. Your body deserves better than a quick fix; it deserves a sustainable path to lasting relief.

Shifting the Paradigm: Embracing Real Solutions Over Temporary Fixes

The pursuit of pain relief often leads us down a winding path, filled with promises of quick fixes and temporary reprieves. But what if we told you that true healing requires a shift in perspective – a move away from simply masking symptoms and towards addressing the root cause of your discomfort?

The Band-Aid Approach: Unmasking the Trap of Temporary Relief

Think of a leaky pipe in your basement. You could simply mop up the water each time it spills, addressing the immediate issue. However, a more effective solution would be to identify the source of the leak and repair it permanently. This principle applies directly to pain management.

While painkillers, injections, or other temporary solutions may offer temporary relief, they rarely address the root cause of your discomfort. This "band-aid" approach might provide short-term comfort but often creates a cycle of dependence, increased dosage, and potentially serious side effects without addressing the underlying issue.

This isn't to say that temporary pain management is always detrimental. There are situations, like after an acute injury or surgery, where short-term relief is necessary. But even then, it's crucial to use these measures judiciously as part of a comprehensive plan that targets the root cause of your pain.

A Slippery Slope: Dependency and the Price of Prolonged Pain Relief

Our bodies are amazing at adapting, but sometimes that adaptability can backfire, especially when it comes to managing pain. We might find relief initially from medications or therapies, but our bodies can become accustomed to them, like old friends showing up at every party, leading to reliance – both physically and mentally.

Think of it this way: physical dependence is like your body becoming a bit of a diva. It gets used to a substance, gets comfy with it, and then demands its daily dose just to function "normally." Suddenly, stopping cold turkey can feel like missing your morning coffee – withdrawal symptoms like increased pain, nausea, anxiety, or sleepless nights start making themselves known.

Then there's psychological dependence, where the emotional connection with the substance kicks in. You start to feel like you can't cope with your pain or even function without it, like a security blanket you can't live without. This can lead to cravings, constant thoughts about getting your fix, and struggles to keep your usage in check.

Opioids, while necessary sometimes to handle extreme, short-term pain, have a reputation for being a bit like that bad friend who's always tempting you. They're notorious for their addictive potential. Long-term use can lead to tolerance (needing higher and higher doses for the same effect), dependence, and, in some cases, addiction – a chronic brain disease where the substance takes over your life, leading to obsessive cravings and use, even when it's causing harm.

Beyond the risk of dependence, many pain management methods have their own list of potential downsides. NSAID pain relievers, for instance, can increase the risk of stomach bleeding, kidney issues, and even heart problems. Opioids can make you sleepy, cause constipation, nausea, slowed breathing, and even affect your thinking. And invasive procedures like injections or surgery always come with the risk of infections, nerve damage, and even chronic pain.

The bottom line is this: it's crucial to weigh the potential benefits of any pain management approach against its risks. Always explore alternative, non-medicinal options whenever possible. Remember, your body is a complex, amazing thing, and taking care of it is always worth the effort.

A Diminishing Return: The Challenge of Tolerance

You know how sometimes a remedy just stops working as well as it used to? That's tolerance in action. Your body gets used to a medication or therapy, and it needs a bigger dose to get the same effect. This is a real headache, especially with pain management.

Think about it: if you rely solely on masking the pain, your body might just learn to live with the medication, making it less effective over time. It's like a slippery slope – you need more and more, increasing the chances of side effects, and eventually, you might need something even stronger.

That's why understanding tolerance is key. It empowers you to make smarter choices about your pain. Instead of just covering up the symptoms, try to figure out what's causing the pain in the first place. Explore different treatments – a mix of approaches might be the ticket to lasting relief without falling into the tolerance trap.

Trapped in a Loop: Breaking Free from the Cycle of Pain Management

For many individuals with chronic pain, the pursuit of relief becomes a cyclical journey - a seemingly endless loop of seeking quick fixes, experiencing temporary relief, encountering side effects or tolerance, and ultimately needing stronger or more frequent interventions. This cycle can be physically and emotionally draining, leaving individuals feeling like they're at the mercy of their pain, their lives dictated by doctor's appointments, medication schedules, and the fear of flare-ups.

Here's how this cycle often unfolds:

1. **Pain Flares:** You experience a surge of pain, disrupting your life and triggering a sense of urgency to find relief.
2. **Seeking a Quick Fix:** You reach for the most readily available solution – typically pain medication, leading to temporary relief but not addressing the underlying issue.
3. **Temporary Relief, Masking the Problem:** The pain subsides, and you feel a sense of hope. However, because the root cause remains unaddressed, the pain inevitably returns.
4. **Escalating Dosages and Interventions:** As your body adapts to the initial treatment, you might find yourself needing higher doses or more

frequent interventions (stronger medications, more frequent injections, etc.) to achieve the same level of relief.

5. **Side Effects and Dependence:** Prolonged use of pain medications or reliance on certain therapies can lead to unwanted side effects, tolerance (needing higher doses for the same effect), or even dependence, both physical and psychological.

6. **Frustration and Despair:** As the cycle repeats, you might feel frustrated, hopeless, and trapped in a system that doesn't seem to offer lasting solutions.

This cycle highlights the limitations of pain *management* and underscores the need for pain *resolution* – a shift from simply masking symptoms to addressing the root cause and empowering individuals with the tools and strategies to regain control of their health.

Taking Back Control: Navigating Your Pain Relief Options With Confidence

In the complex and often confusing world of pain management, knowledge is your most powerful ally. By becoming an informed advocate for your own health, you can make empowered choices that align with your values, goals, and long-term well-being.

Becoming Your Own Health Detective: The Power of Self-Education

In today's digital age, we have access to an overwhelming amount of information at our fingertips. While this can be both a blessing and a curse, it also presents an unprecedented opportunity to become informed healthcare consumers.

Here are a few tips for effectively educating yourself about pain management options:

- **Start with Reliable Sources:** Look for information from reputable organizations, such as the National Institutes of Health (NIH), the Mayo Clinic, or the Cleveland Clinic. Be wary of websites selling products or promoting quick fixes.
- **Dive Deeper into Research:** If you encounter a treatment or therapy that piques your interest, explore the research behind it. Look for studies published in peer-reviewed medical journals that involve a significant number of participants and utilize rigorous scientific methods.
- **Be Critical of Testimonials:** While personal stories can be inspiring, it's important to remember that individual experiences can vary widely. Testimonials should not be mistaken for scientific evidence.

- **Join Support Groups and Online Communities:** Connect with others who are navigating similar health challenges. These communities can provide valuable insights, emotional support, and practical tips for managing pain.

Engaging in Meaningful Dialogue: Questions to Ask Your Doctor

Open, honest communication with your healthcare providers is essential for receiving the best possible care. Don't be afraid to advocate for your needs, ask questions, and express your concerns. Remember, you are an active participant in your healing journey, and your voice matters.

Here are some key questions to ask your doctor about pain management options:

- **What is the root cause of my pain?** (Don't settle for "It's just arthritis" or "It's because you're getting older.")
- **What are the potential benefits and risks of this treatment?**
- **Are there any alternative therapies or lifestyle changes I can try?**
- **What can I expect in terms of recovery time and potential side effects?**

- **How long will I need to be on this medication?**
(Especially if you're prescribed pain relievers)
- **What are the long-term implications of this treatment approach?**
- **What happens if this treatment doesn't work?**

By asking these questions, you'll gain a deeper understanding of your condition, the proposed treatments, and potential alternatives. This will empower you to make informed decisions about your health and actively participate in creating a pain management plan that aligns with your values and goals.

Finding Your Voice: Becoming an Advocate for Your Health

In the realm of healthcare, it's easy to slip into a passive role, deferring to doctors and accepting treatments without fully understanding the risks, benefits, or alternatives. But remember, this is *your* body, *your* health, and *your* life. You have the right to be an active participant in your care, to ask questions, express concerns, and advocate for your needs.

Here are a few tips for effectively advocating for your health:

- **Come Prepared:** Before appointments, write down your questions, concerns, and goals. This will help you stay focused and ensure that you cover everything you need to discuss with your doctor.

- **Bring an Advocate:** If you feel overwhelmed or intimidated in medical settings, bring a trusted friend or family member to appointments for support. Having someone by your side can make it easier to ask questions, remember information, and advocate for your needs.

- **Don't Be Afraid to Seek Second Opinions:** If you're unsure about a diagnosis, treatment recommendation, or prognosis, don't hesitate to seek a second opinion from another qualified healthcare professional. You have the right to gather information from multiple sources before making decisions about your health.

- **Trust Your Instincts:** You know your body better than anyone. If something doesn't feel right, if a treatment doesn't seem to be working, or if you have concerns about potential side effects, speak up! Your voice matters.

Weighing the Options: Making Informed Decisions for Your Well-Being

Making decisions about your health, especially when it comes to pain management, can feel overwhelming. But by arming yourself with knowledge, advocating for your needs, and exploring a variety of options, you can confidently choose a path that aligns with your values, priorities, and long-term health goals.

Here's a framework to guide your decision-making process:

1. **Gather Information:** Research your condition, explore different treatment options, understand the potential benefits and risks, and consider the long-term implications of each choice.
2. **Seek Professional Guidance:** Consult with qualified healthcare providers who align with your values and prioritize a holistic approach. Ask questions, express your concerns, and don't be afraid to seek second opinions.
3. **Tune into Your Intuition:** Your body is incredibly wise. Pay attention to how you feel physically and emotionally as you consider different options. What resonates with you? What feels aligned with your intuition?
4. **Consider Your Lifestyle and Preferences:** Choose treatments and therapies that fit within your lifestyle, values, and preferences. There's no one-size-fits-all approach to healing.
5. **Be Patient and Flexible:** Healing is a journey, not a race. Be patient with yourself, allow for setbacks, and be willing to adjust your approach as needed.

You are the CEO of your own body. By embracing your role as an informed and empowered healthcare consumer, you can confidently navigate the world of pain management options, ask the right questions, and make choices that support your long-term health and well-being.

ACTION STEP: Learn the 3 secrets to reversing spine and joint pain by scanning the code below.

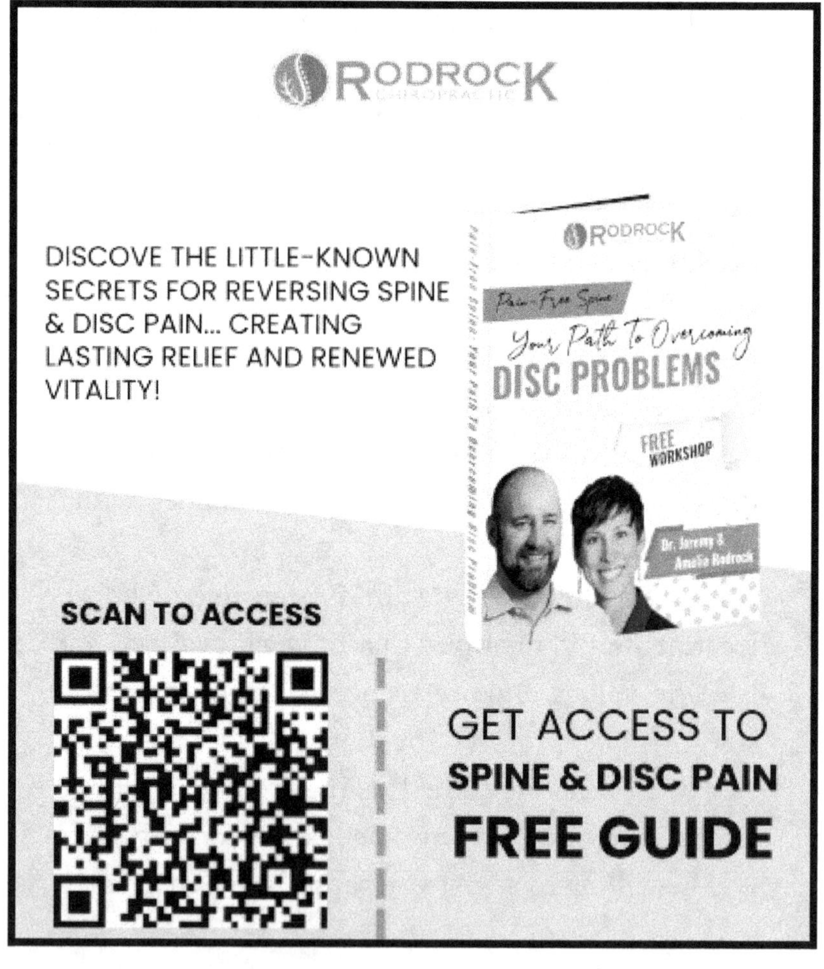

Jennifer's Rave Review of Rodrock Chiropractic

"Everything about Rodrock Chiropractic is exceptional. From the waiting area, office staff, chiropractors, and massage therapists. Everyone is friendly, professional, and knowledgeable. You feel like family on the first visit. My daughter and I have had great success with treatments, and I'm so glad they are right here in Baldwin City."

Feel like yourself again. Call 785-465-5605 to take the first step in reversing your pain and regaining your freedom.

** Individual results may vary. Please review the disclaimer after the Table of Contents.*

4

BEYOND THE MISCONCEPTIONS: UNVEILING COMMON MYTHS AND MISTAKES ABOUT PAIN

We've all grown up with certain beliefs about pain – some helpful, some harmful, and many simply misguided. These ingrained beliefs, often shaped by cultural norms, personal experiences, or misinformation, can profoundly influence how we perceive, respond to, and ultimately manage pain.

This chapter explores common myths and mistakes surrounding pain, particularly spine and joint pain. By dispelling these misconceptions, we empower you to develop a more accurate and empowering understanding of your body's signals and make informed choices that support your healing journey.

Reframing the Narrative: Moving from Fear to Understanding

One of the most pervasive misconceptions about pain is that it's something to be feared, avoided, and silenced at all costs. We're conditioned to view pain as an enemy – an unwelcome intruder that disrupts our lives and limits our potential. But what if we told you that pain, in its purest form, is actually a messenger, a vital part of your body's intricate communication system?

Pain as a Protector: Understanding Your Body's Warning System

Imagine this: you accidentally touch a hot stove. Instantly, pain receptors in your hand send a message to your brain, triggering a lightning-fast withdrawal reflex that prevents a severe burn. In this scenario, pain isn't the enemy; it's your protector, a vital messenger alerting you to danger and prompting you to take action to prevent further harm.

While chronic pain is far more complex than this simple example, the underlying principle remains the same. Pain, even when persistent, is often your body's way of signaling that something is amiss, that something needs attention. It might be a misalignment in your spine, inflammation in a joint, a muscle imbalance, or even chronic stress that's manifesting physically.

Tuning Out the Body: The Perils of Ignoring Pain Signals

We're masters at brushing off those nagging little aches and pains. "Just a bit stiff," we mutter, or "a touch sore, it'll pass." We push through the discomfort, chalking it up to the wear and tear of life, the inevitable march of time, or even a sign of weakness. But what if those whispers of discomfort are our body's way of shouting for help?

Think of it like your car's dashboard. That little light flickering insistently? You might initially ignore it, hoping it's nothing serious. But if it keeps blinking, it's a clear signal that something's amiss under the hood. Ignoring those warning signs can lead to a complete breakdown, leaving you stranded and frustrated.

Our bodies are no different. Persistent pain isn't some badge of honor; it's a plea for attention. Ignoring it won't make it vanish. Instead, it often festers, growing into something more serious, robbing us of mobility and increasing the risk of complications.

The Invisible Burden: Addressing the Stigma of Chronic Pain

Many individuals with chronic pain, particularly those dealing with conditions that aren't readily visible or easily understood, often face a sense of isolation and stigma. The world doesn't always see their struggles, and their pain can be dismissed as "all in their head" or a sign of weakness.

Here's why the stigma surrounding chronic pain is so harmful:

- **It silences the voice of those who suffer:** Individuals with chronic pain might feel like they can't talk about their struggles, fear being judged, or worry about being dismissed.
- **It perpetuates misconceptions about pain:** The stigma often reinforces the myth that pain is a psychological issue, not a physical reality.
- **It hinders access to proper care:** Individuals who feel stigmatized might be reluctant to seek help or be hesitant to openly communicate their needs with healthcare providers.

Breaking the stigma surrounding chronic pain requires empathy, understanding, and a willingness to listen. It's about recognizing that pain, whether visible or invisible, is real, impacting people's lives in profound ways.

The Labyrinth of Misdiagnosis: Navigating the Challenges of Pain Management

Imagine seeking help for a persistent cough and being told it's just a cold, only to discover weeks later that you have pneumonia. Or, imagine going to the doctor with back pain and being prescribed pain relievers without a thorough assessment of the underlying cause. These scenarios illustrate the challenges of navigating the complex world of pain management.

Here are some common reasons for misdiagnosis and mismanagement of pain:

- **Limited Time with Healthcare Providers:** The fast-paced nature of modern healthcare often leaves little time for comprehensive assessments and open dialogue between patients and doctors. This can lead to hasty diagnoses, overlooking potential underlying conditions or neglecting to explore a full range of treatment options.
- **Overreliance on Imaging:** While imaging studies like X-rays or MRIs can be helpful in identifying structural problems, they often fail to capture the full picture of pain. Soft tissue injuries, nerve compression, and other factors can contribute to pain, but these may not be visible on imaging studies.
- **Lack of Understanding About Pain Mechanisms:** Pain is a complex phenomenon, involving a symphony of neural, hormonal, and psychological factors. A lack of understanding about these mechanisms can lead to misdiagnosis, inappropriate treatment choices, and a cycle of persistent pain.
- **Stigma and Misconceptions:** The stigma surrounding chronic pain can make it difficult for

individuals to openly communicate their experiences, leading to misdiagnosis or a lack of empathy from healthcare providers.

The good news is that awareness of these challenges can empower you to take control of your health. Be an active participant in your care, ask questions, seek second opinions if you're unsure, and don't be afraid to advocate for your needs. Remember, you are the expert on your own body.

Reclaiming Your Movement: Unmasking Lifestyle Pitfalls That Fuel Pain

We often attribute pain to aging, genetics, or unavoidable injuries, but the truth is that many cases of spine and joint pain are fueled by our modern lifestyle choices. These seemingly insignificant habits, often overlooked in the pursuit of convenience and efficiency, can unknowingly contribute to chronic discomfort, limited mobility, and a decline in overall health.

The Sedentary Lifestyle: A Modern Trap for Spine and Joint Health

Our modern world is designed for convenience, rewarding us for minimizing movement and maximizing efficiency. We drive instead of walk, take the elevator instead of the stairs, and spend hours glued to our desks or screens. While these choices might save us time in the short term, they can have detrimental effects on our spine and joints over time.

Here's why a sedentary lifestyle can contribute to pain:

- **Muscle Weakness and Imbalances:** Without regular movement, our muscles weaken and become imbalanced. This can lead to poor posture, strain on joints, and increased risk of injury.
- **Decreased Joint Lubrication:** Movement helps to circulate synovial fluid, the lubricant that cushions and protects your joints. A sedentary lifestyle can lead to decreased joint lubrication, increasing friction and wear and tear, which can ultimately contribute to pain and stiffness.
- **Reduced Blood Flow:** Movement promotes blood circulation, delivering oxygen and nutrients to your tissues. When you're sedentary for prolonged periods, blood flow can stagnate, potentially leading to inflammation and pain.
- **Increased Stress:** When we're inactive, our bodies tend to hold more tension, which can contribute to muscle tightness, stiffness, and pain.

Breaking free from the sedentary trap doesn't require a radical overhaul; it's about incorporating small, consistent changes into your daily routine. Start by taking the stairs instead of the elevator, parking a little further away from the entrance, taking walking breaks during the workday, or engaging in gentle exercises that promote movement and flexibility.

Fueling the Fire: How Diet Choices Can Contribute to Spine and Joint Pain

We're often told "you are what you eat," and this adage rings especially true when it comes to spine and joint health. Just as a car needs high-quality fuel to run smoothly, our bodies rely on a balanced, nutrient-rich diet to function at their best and to repair and protect our delicate joints.

Here's how poor diet choices can contribute to spine and joint pain:

- **The Inflammation Connection:** Certain foods, particularly processed foods, sugary drinks, and unhealthy fats, trigger an inflammatory response in the body. This inflammation can contribute to pain, stiffness, and accelerated wear and tear on your joints.
- **Nutritional Deficiencies:** A lack of essential nutrients, such as calcium, vitamin D, omega-3 fatty acids, and collagen, can compromise bone density, joint lubrication, and tissue repair, ultimately increasing your susceptibility to pain.
- **Gut Health and Inflammation:** The health of your

gut microbiome – the trillions of bacteria that live in your digestive system – plays a crucial role in overall health, including your immune system and inflammatory response. An unhealthy gut can lead to increased inflammation throughout the body, contributing to pain and stiffness.

- **Weight Management:** Excess weight places additional stress on your spine and joints, making them more vulnerable to injury and pain.

Making mindful food choices can be a powerful tool for managing spine and joint pain. Here are a few tips:

- **Prioritize Whole, Unprocessed Foods:** Focus on fruits, vegetables, whole grains, lean protein, and healthy fats.
- **Hydrate Regularly:** Water is essential for joint lubrication and overall health.
- **Limit Processed Foods, Sugary Drinks, and Unhealthy Fats:** These foods contribute to inflammation and can exacerbate pain.
- **Consider Supplements:** Talk to your healthcare provider about potential supplements that might support your spine and joint health, such as omega-3 fatty acids, vitamin D, and collagen.
- **Mindful Eating:** Pay attention to how different foods make you feel.

What you eat is a powerful tool for supporting your body's natural healing abilities and reducing your risk of pain.

The Silent Saboteur: How Stress and Sleep Deprivation Fuel Pain

We often think of stress and sleep deprivation as primarily impacting our mood and mental well-being, but they also have a profound impact on our physical health, particularly our spine and joints.

Here's how stress and sleeplessness can contribute to pain:

- **Stress Hormones:** When we're stressed, our bodies release hormones like cortisol and adrenaline. These hormones, while helpful in short bursts, can contribute to chronic inflammation, muscle tension, and even altered pain perception when experienced chronically.
- **Muscle Tension:** Stress can lead to chronic muscle tension, especially in the neck, shoulders, and back. This tension can create pain, reduce mobility, and increase your susceptibility to injury.
- **Sleep Deprivation:** When we don't get enough restorative sleep, our bodies don't have time to repair and rebuild tissues, leading to increased inflammation, heightened pain perception, and a weakened immune system.
- **Increased Pain Sensitivity:** Lack of sleep can

make us more sensitive to pain signals, making even minor aches and stiffness feel more intense.

Here are a few tips for managing stress and improving sleep quality:

- **Practice Mindfulness and Relaxation Techniques:** Engage in activities that help you de-stress, such as deep breathing exercises, meditation, yoga, or spending time in nature.
- **Establish a Regular Sleep Routine:** Go to bed and wake up around the same time each day, even on weekends, to regulate your body's natural sleep-wake cycle.
- **Create a Conducive Sleep Environment:** Ensure a dark, quiet, and cool sleep space, and avoid screen time an hour before bed.
- **Limit Caffeine and Alcohol:** These substances can interfere with sleep.
- **Get Regular Exercise:** Physical activity can help reduce stress and promote better sleep.
- **Seek Professional Help:** If you're struggling with chronic stress or sleep issues, reach out to a qualified healthcare professional for personalized guidance and support.

Taking care of your mental and emotional well-being is essential for supporting your physical health.

Beyond the Conventional: Breaking Free from Healing Hurdles

It's understandable to seek quick fixes and rely on conventional approaches when dealing with pain. But the path to lasting relief often requires a shift in perspective—an embrace of holistic methods that consider the interconnectedness of your body, mind, and spirit.

The Narrow Focus: Overlooking the Benefits of a Holistic Approach

The body, a symphony of interconnected systems, whispers its pain in a language often misunderstood. While the conventional approach seeks to silence the discordant notes with medication and intervention, it sometimes overlooks the melody's deeper harmony.

Chronic pain, a persistent ache that lingers long after the initial wound has healed, is rarely a solitary note. It's a complex composition, woven from threads of postural imbalances, muscle weakness, dietary deficiencies, the relentless rhythm of stress, and the unspoken melodies of emotional distress.

A holistic approach listens intently to the body's symphony, recognizing that true healing lies not in silencing the pain but in understanding its intricate composition. It seeks to restore balance, harmonize the discordant notes, and allow the body's innate wisdom to guide the path towards wholeness.

The Uniqueness of Healing: Rejecting the One-Size-Fits-All Fallacy

There's a certain vulnerability that comes with receiving medical advice. We place our trust in the hands of experts, hoping for relief, for answers. Yet, sometimes the prescribed path feels discordant, a melody out of tune with our own inner rhythm.

Pain management, like life itself, resists easy categorization. It's not a one-size-fits-all equation. Just as our fingerprints are unique, so too are our experiences of pain, our bodies' responses, and the tapestry of factors that contribute to our well-being.

What brings solace to one soul might leave another feeling lost. A treatment that works today might lose its efficacy tomorrow. True healing, then, becomes a journey of self-discovery, a delicate dance between expert guidance and personal intuition. It's about honoring the individual narrative, the unique symphony that plays within each of us.

The Art of Patience: Embracing the Journey of Healing

Healing from chronic pain, particularly when it's become a persistent part of your life, takes time, patience, and a willingness to embrace the process. It's not about striving for perfection or expecting rapid, dramatic results. It's about making consistent, positive changes, celebrating small victories, and staying committed to your long-term goals.

Here are a few tips for cultivating patience on your healing journey:

- **Shift Your Mindset:** Focus on progress, not perfection. Celebrate every step forward, even if it feels small.
- **Track Your Progress:** Keeping a pain journal or using a pain tracking app can help you monitor your progress, identify triggers, and adjust your approach as needed.
- **Be Kind to Yourself:** Healing takes time, and setbacks are inevitable. Allow yourself grace, and don't be discouraged if you encounter challenges along the way.
- **Seek Support:** Connect with healthcare providers who understand your journey, with support groups, or with loved ones who can offer encouragement and understanding.

Dealing with pain can feel like climbing a mountain, especially when you're bombarded with conflicting advice, limited options, and the pressure to feel better right now. But remember, your body isn't a machine; it's a complex and beautiful symphony of interconnected systems. True healing takes time and a gentle, holistic approach. It's about understanding the unique story your pain is telling, digging deep to find the root cause, and treating your whole self – mind, body, and spirit.

Let go of the idea of quick fixes and embrace a path that's tailored just for you. Be patient with yourself, celebrate small victories, and remember that lasting relief is possible. Imagine a life filled with movement, vitality, and joy – that's the destination waiting for you on this journey.

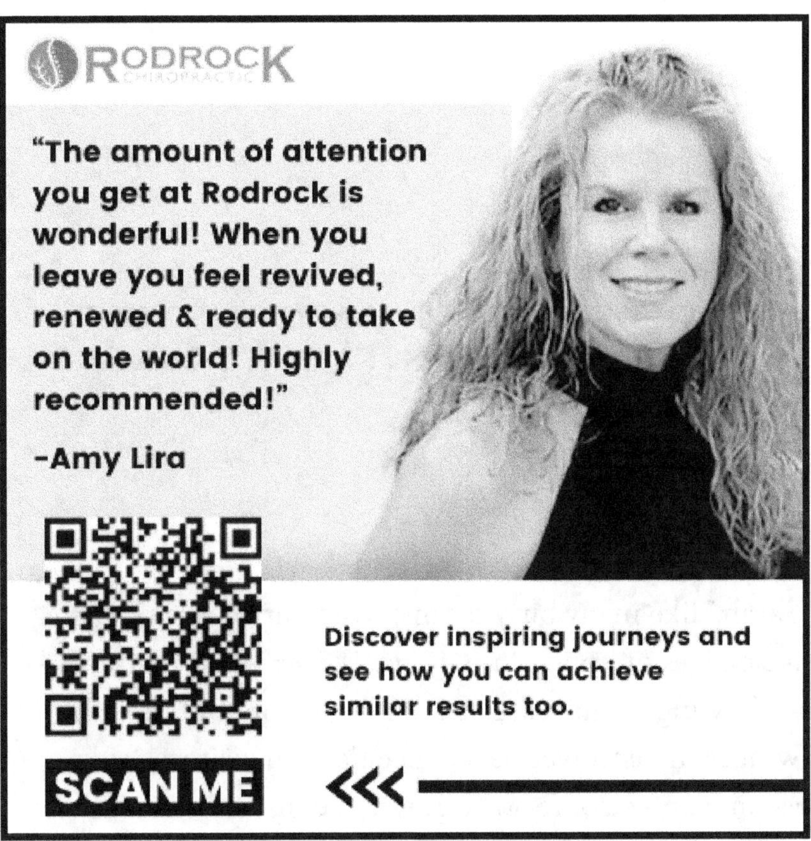

Don't wait for pain to get worse – call 785-465-5605 and reclaim your comfort and mobility today.

** Individual results may vary. Please review the disclaimer after the Table of Contents.*

5

EARLY SIGNS AND SYMPTOMS YOUR BODY DOESN'T WANT YOU TO IGNORE

"Sarah," like many busy moms, wore her aches and pains like badges of honor. *'Just lifting the kids,'* she'd mutter, swallowing a painkiller and soldiering on. But those little twinges in her lower back, once fleeting visitors, had become unwelcome houseguests, a constant ache that snaked down her leg. What started as a minor inconvenience, a whisper of discomfort easily ignored, had blossomed into a full-blown herniated disc, demanding surgery and months of grueling rehab.

Sarah's story is a stark reminder that our bodies are constantly trying to communicate with us. Those subtle aches, the stiffness that lingers a little too long, the twinges that make us wince – they're not just the price we pay for a hectic life. They're whispers, sometimes urgent, sometimes gentle, begging us to slow down, to listen, to address the root cause before a minor issue explodes into a major crisis.

Decoding the Messages: Understanding Your Body's Language

Our bodies are incredibly complex systems, constantly communicating with us through a language of sensations. Learning to understand this language, to distinguish between transient discomfort and persistent warnings, is essential for maintaining well-being and preventing more serious issues.

One key distinction is between acute and chronic pain. Acute pain is a sudden, sharp signal, alerting us to immediate injury or threat. Think of a sprained ankle, a burn, or a cut – the pain is intense but typically subsides as the body heals.

Chronic pain, however, is a more insidious foe. It's a persistent ache that lingers long after the initial injury has healed, often lasting for months or even years. This can be due to a variety of factors, including inflammation, joint degeneration, nerve compression, muscle imbalances, or even unresolved emotional stress.

It's important to remember that even seemingly minor aches or stiffness that recur regularly should not be ignored. These recurring whispers of discomfort can be your body's way of signaling a deeper imbalance or dysfunction that requires attention.

By paying attention to our body's signals and seeking appropriate care when needed, we can foster a deeper connection with ourselves and promote long-term health and well-being.

Your Body, a Finely Tuned Machine: The Importance of Early Detection

Imagine your body as a finely tuned machine, like a high-performance car. Just as a car needs regular maintenance, oil changes, and prompt attention to any unusual noises or warning lights, so too does your body require care, attention, and early intervention to prevent minor issues from escalating into major breakdowns.

Ignoring those subtle knocks, rattles, or warning lights in your car might seem harmless in the short term, but over time, they can lead to costly repairs, decreased performance, and even dangerous breakdowns. Similarly, dismissing those persistent aches, stiffness, or limited range of motion in your body can have far-reaching consequences, ultimately impacting your mobility, your overall health, and your quality of life.

Early intervention is key. Just as addressing a minor engine issue can prevent major engine failure, addressing those early signs of pain and dysfunction can prevent chronic pain, mobility limitations, and the need for more invasive interventions down the road.

Recognizing the Red Flags: Early Warning Signs You Shouldn't Ignore

Your body has a remarkable way of communicating its needs, often sending subtle signals long before a minor ache escalates into a debilitating condition. Learning to recognize these early warning signs empowers you to take action, seek timely intervention, and potentially prevent more serious problems down the road.

Here are some common red flags for back, neck, and joint pain that warrant attention:

Back Pain Red Flags:

- **Pain that intensifies at night or disrupts your sleep.** While some discomfort is normal, pain that worsens when you lie down or prevents you from getting a good night's sleep could signal a more serious issue, such as a herniated disc or spinal stenosis.
- **Pain that travels down your leg or arm.** This radiating pain, often accompanied by numbness, tingling, or weakness, could indicate nerve compression or irritation, such as sciatica (pain

radiating down the leg) or cervical radiculopathy (pain radiating down the arm).

- **Numbness, tingling, or weakness in your limbs.** These neurological symptoms can indicate nerve compression or damage, requiring prompt attention.
- **Loss of bladder or bowel control.** This is a medical emergency and requires immediate attention.

Neck Pain Signals:

- **Frequent headaches, especially at the base of your skull.** Tension headaches are common, but headaches that originate in the back of the head and neck or are accompanied by neck stiffness or pain could indicate underlying neck dysfunction.
- **Pain that worsens with prolonged sitting or computer use.** Poor posture, especially when combined with prolonged sitting, can strain neck muscles and joints, leading to pain and stiffness.
- **Stiffness that limits your ability to turn your head.** This could indicate joint restriction, muscle tightness, or other underlying issues in the neck.
- **Pain that travels down your shoulders or arms.** Similar to radiating back pain, this type of pain could signal nerve compression in the neck.

Joint Pain Clues:

- **Morning stiffness and pain that gradually improve with movement.** While some morning stiffness is normal, prolonged stiffness that lasts for more than 30 minutes or interferes with daily activities could indicate inflammatory conditions like arthritis.

- **Clicking, popping, or grinding sounds with movement.** These sounds, while not always a cause for concern, can sometimes indicate joint instability, cartilage damage, or other underlying issues.

- **Swelling or warmth around the joint.** These signs often indicate inflammation, which could be a result of injury, overuse, or underlying inflammatory conditions.

- **Limited range of motion or difficulty performing daily tasks.** If you're experiencing difficulty with everyday activities like walking, climbing stairs, gripping objects, or turning your head, it's essential to seek professional guidance to address the underlying cause of your limitations.

Taking Charge: The Power of Early Intervention for Spine and Joint Health

The adage "an ounce of prevention is worth a pound of cure" rings true when it comes to spine and joint health. Seeking help sooner rather than later is not a sign of weakness; it's a courageous act of self-care, a proactive approach to preventing minor issues from escalating into major problems.

Here are some key benefits of early intervention:

- **Increased Chances of Faster, More Complete Healing:** When addressed early, many spine and joint problems respond well to conservative treatments, such as chiropractic adjustments, physical therapy, massage therapy, and lifestyle modifications. These approaches focus on restoring proper joint mechanics, reducing inflammation, improving muscle strength and flexibility, and addressing underlying contributing factors. Early intervention can often prevent the need for more invasive procedures like injections or surgery.
- **Potential for Avoiding Invasive Procedures or Long-Term Medication Reliance:** The sooner you address pain and dysfunction, the greater the chances of avoiding a cascade of interventions, including injections, surgery, or long-term pain

medication reliance. Early intervention often allows for a gentler, more natural healing process, reducing the risk of side effects, dependence, and complications associated with more invasive treatments.

- **Maintaining Mobility, Independence, and Quality of Life:** Ignoring persistent pain often leads to a cycle of decline, with gradually diminishing mobility, increasing limitations in daily activities, and a reduced quality of life. Early intervention can help prevent this downward spiral, allowing you to maintain your independence, participate in activities you enjoy, and live life to the fullest.

- **Reduced Risk of Chronic Pain:** Many pain conditions become chronic because they're left unaddressed for prolonged periods. Early intervention can help prevent the transition from acute to chronic pain, potentially avoiding the more complex and challenging aspects of managing chronic pain syndromes.

- **Improved Long-Term Health Outcomes:** Taking proactive steps to address pain and dysfunction can have a positive impact on your overall health and well-being, not just your spine and joints. Early intervention often leads to improved posture, better balance, increased muscle strength and flexibility, and a reduced risk of future injuries or conditions.

Don't wait for pain to become debilitating. Trust your body's signals, seek help early, and create a future where you move freely and live life to the fullest.

Taking Action: Your Next Steps Toward a Pain-Free Life

Recognizing early signs of pain and dysfunction is a crucial first step, but it's just the beginning. Now, it's time to take action and empower yourself to reclaim your health and well-being.

Here are some practical steps you can take right now:

- **Schedule a Consultation with Us:** We're here to listen, understand your unique story, and help you develop a personalized plan for pain relief and lasting wellness. You can schedule an appointment by visiting our website, <u>https://chirorock.-com/contact/</u>, or contacting our Lawrence office or Baldwin City office at 785-465-5605. Please note that scheduling a consultation does not guarantee specific results. Every individual's condition and response to treatment varies.
- **Start a Pain Journal:** Tracking your pain can be a powerful tool for understanding its patterns, identifying triggers, and measuring progress. Consider creating a journal where you record:

- The location, intensity, and duration of your pain
- Activities or events that seem to worsen or alleviate your pain
- Any medications or treatments you've tried and their effectiveness
- Your overall mood, energy levels, and sleep quality
- Your progress over time
- **Incorporate Gentle Movement and Stretches:** Regular movement is essential for maintaining joint health, reducing muscle tension, and improving blood circulation. Even simple stretches and light exercises can make a big difference in your overall comfort and well-being. Start with a few gentle stretches each day, and gradually increase the intensity and duration as you feel more comfortable.

Every step you take towards understanding your body, seeking help, and making positive changes is a step towards a pain-free, vibrant life. We're here to support you on this journey.

Reclaiming Your Power: Embracing a Future Free From Pain

We understand that the journey to pain relief can feel daunting, but we want to remind you that you don't have to be a victim of your pain. You have the power to make choices that support your health, to break free from the limitations of chronic discomfort, and to create a life filled with movement, vitality, and joy.

The RESTORE Framework empowers you to take control of your well-being, to become an active participant in your healing journey, and to embrace a future free from pain. It's about understanding your body's signals, seeking guidance from trusted professionals, and making choices that align with your values and goals.

It's about listening to your body, recognizing those early whispers of discomfort, and taking action before minor issues escalate into major problems. It's about becoming your own advocate, asking questions, seeking second opinions, and actively participating in your care.

It's about embracing the power of a holistic approach, understanding that true healing involves addressing the physical, emotional, and lifestyle factors that contribute to your pain.

It's about trusting in your body's innate healing abilities and giving it the support it needs to thrive.

It's about reclaiming your life, one step at a time.

Ready to embark on your journey toward lasting relief? Contact us today to learn more about the RESTORE Framework and schedule a consultation. You can reach our Baldwin City office or Lawrence office at 785-465-

5605. You can also schedule an appointment or learn more by visiting our website at https://chirorock.com/contact/. We're here to support you every step of the way. Please note that a consultation does not guarantee specific results as individual conditions and responses to treatment can vary.

ACTION STEP: Scan the code below to download our 25 Anti-Inflammatory Recipes Guide.

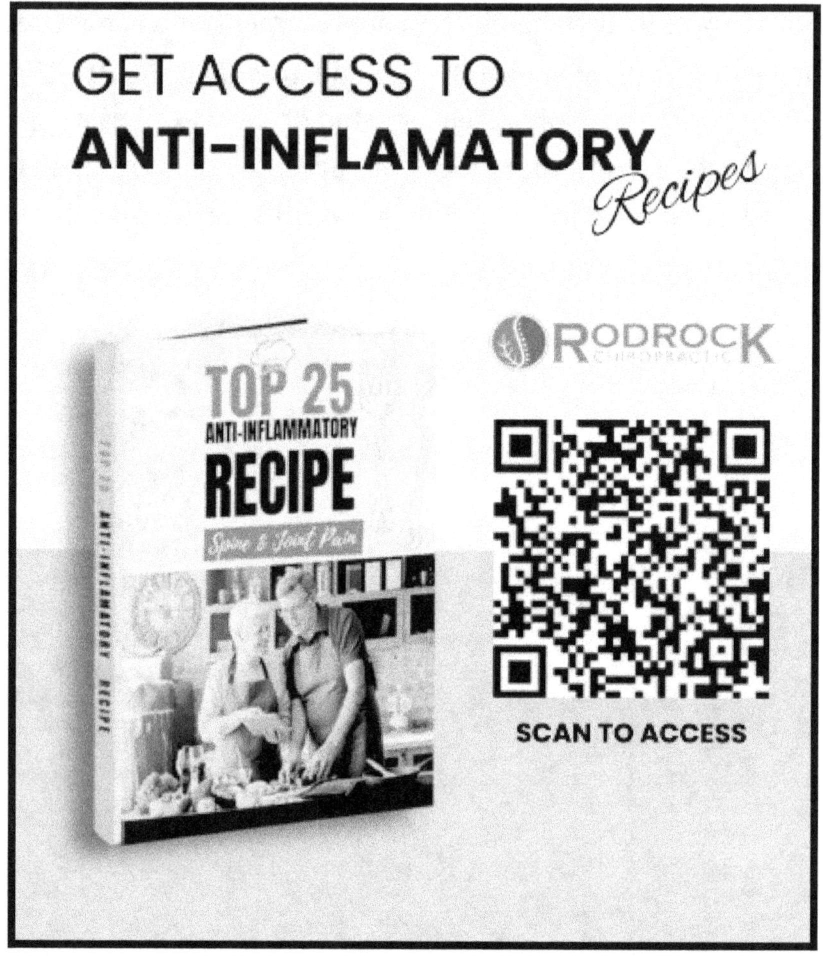

Cathy's Relief: Migraines, Headaches, and Back Pain Gone

"I've been seeing Dr. Jeremy for many years. I suffered from migraines, headaches, and back pain. Getting regular adjustments has helped tremendously! He's always nice and gentle with my five-year-old daughter as well as all the office staff."

Your relief starts here. Call 785-465-5605 now to get personalized care for your back and neck pain.

** Individual results may vary. Please review the disclaimer after the Table of Contents.*

** Every patient's journey is unique. This testimonial does not guarantee similar results for others.*

6

THE FOOD-SPINE CONNECTION: NOURISHING YOUR WAY TO A HEALTHIER BACK

Imagine your spine as a majestic oak tree, its roots anchoring it deep within the earth, its trunk providing strength and stability, its branches reaching towards the sky. Just as a tree relies on nutrient-rich soil to thrive, your spine depends on the nourishment you provide through your diet to stay strong, flexible, and resilient.

For far too long, we've separated the act of eating from its profound impact on our musculoskeletal health. But the truth is, the food on your plate can either nourish and protect your spine or contribute to inflammation, stiffness, and accelerated wear and tear. This chapter explores the powerful connection between nutrition and spinal health, revealing how making conscious food choices can be a delicious and empowering act of self-care for your back.

The Double-Edged Sword of Inflammation: Friend or Foe?

We often hear "inflammation" and immediately picture swollen joints and throbbing pain. It's true, chronic inflammation can be a real troublemaker, contributing to conditions like arthritis and even degenerative disc disease. But here's the thing: inflammation isn't always the villain.

Think of it like your body's own internal alarm system. When you twist your ankle, cut your finger, or even experience irritation in your spine, inflammation kicks in. It's like a rush of healing superheroes, rushing to the scene to repair damage and fight off any potential invaders.

The tricky part? What we eat plays a huge role in how this alarm system behaves. A diet loaded with processed foods, sugary drinks, and unhealthy fats is like constantly hitting the panic button, leading to low-grade, chronic inflammation that can wear down our joints and tissues over time.

But there's good news! Choosing a diet rich in whole, unprocessed foods, especially those packed with antioxidants and anti-inflammatory compounds, is like giving your body the tools it needs to keep inflammation in check. It's like providing your internal superheroes with the best equipment to protect your joints and support healing.

Eating for a Healthy Spine: Key Nutrients and Their Superpowers

Just as a builder needs the right materials to construct a strong, stable structure, your body relies on specific nutrients to build and maintain a healthy spine. By incorporating these nutritional powerhouses into your diet, you can provide your body with the building blocks it needs for optimal spinal health.

Here are some key nutrients and their remarkable benefits for your back:

- **Calcium & Vitamin D: The Dynamic Duo for Bone Strength:** Calcium is like the steel frame of your spine, providing structure and strength to your bones, while vitamin D acts as the construction manager, ensuring that calcium is properly absorbed and utilized. Together, they play a crucial role in preventing osteoporosis, a condition that weakens bones and makes them more susceptible to fractures.
- **Food Sources:** Dairy products, leafy green vegetables, fortified foods (like plant-based milk alternatives), fatty fish (like salmon and sardines).
- **Sunshine Boost:** Your body can also produce vitamin D with exposure to sunlight.
- **Omega-3 Fatty Acids: The Inflammation Tamers:** These healthy fats, particularly EPA

(eicosapentaenoic acid) and DHA (docosahexaenoic acid), act like firefighters in your body, taming the flames of inflammation that can contribute to joint pain and stiffness.

- **Food Sources:** Fatty fish (salmon, mackerel, tuna, sardines), walnuts, flaxseeds, chia seeds.
- **Supplement Support:** High-quality fish oil or algae-based omega-3 supplements can also be beneficial.
- **Collagen: The Cushion and Glue for Your Joints:** Think of collagen as the springy cartilage that cushions your vertebrae, the strong tendons that connect muscles to bones, and the flexible ligaments that hold your joints together. Collagen provides structural integrity, flexibility, and shock absorption for your spine.
- **Food Sources:** Bone broth, chicken with skin on, fish with skin on, eggs.
- **Supplement Support:** Collagen supplements, particularly hydrolyzed collagen peptides, are easily absorbed and can provide additional support.
- **Antioxidants: The Cellular Protectors:** Just as rust can weaken a metal structure, oxidative stress – an imbalance of free radicals and antioxidants – can damage cells and contribute to aging and disease, including joint degeneration. Antioxidants

found in colorful fruits and vegetables act like rust inhibitors, neutralizing those harmful free radicals and protecting your cells from damage.

- **Food Sources:** A wide variety of colorful fruits and vegetables, such as berries, leafy greens, tomatoes, and citrus fruits. The more vibrant the colors, the higher the antioxidant content!

Building a Back-Friendly Plate: Practical Tips for Everyday Eating

Understanding the science behind nutrition is important, but translating that knowledge into actionable steps is what truly makes a difference. Here are some practical tips to empower you to "eat for a healthy spine" and make food choices that nourish and protect your back:

- **Swap Out Processed for Whole:** Instead of reaching for sugary cereals, white bread, or packaged snacks, opt for whole, unprocessed foods like fruits, vegetables, whole grains, lean proteins, and healthy fats. These nutrient-rich foods provide the building blocks your body needs for optimal spinal health.
- **Embrace Color:** Make your plate a rainbow! The vibrant colors of fruits and vegetables aren't just visually appealing; they reflect a rich diversity of

antioxidants that protect your cells from damage. Aim to include a variety of colorful produce in your meals and snacks.

- **Prioritize Omega-3s:** Make fatty fish (salmon, mackerel, sardines) a regular part of your diet. If you're not a fan of fish, consider incorporating flaxseeds, chia seeds, or walnuts into your meals or talking to your doctor about a high-quality fish oil supplement.
- **Bone Up on Bone Broth:** This savory broth, made from simmering bones, cartilage, and connective tissues, is a source of collagen and other nutrients that support joint health. Enjoy it on its own, use it as a base for soups and stews, or sip on it throughout the day.

Sample Spine-Healthy Meal Ideas:

- **Breakfast:** Oatmeal topped with berries, walnuts, and a sprinkle of flaxseeds; scrambled eggs with spinach and smoked salmon; Greek yogurt with fruit and a drizzle of honey.
- **Lunch:** Large salad with grilled chicken or fish, plenty of colorful veggies, and a light vinaigrette; lentil soup with a side of whole-grain bread; leftovers from dinner!
- **Dinner:** Baked salmon with roasted vegetables; grilled chicken breast with quinoa and steamed

broccoli; lentil and vegetable curry over brown rice.

Hydration Matters:

Don't underestimate the importance of staying hydrated! Water is essential for numerous bodily functions, including transporting nutrients, flushing out waste products, and maintaining the health of your intervertebral discs – the spongy cushions between your vertebrae. Aim to drink plenty of water throughout the day, especially before, during, and after exercise.

Mindful Eating for a Healthy Back:

In our fast-paced world, we often rush through meals, barely paying attention to the food on our plates. But mindful eating – slowing down, savoring each bite, and paying attention to how your body feels – can enhance digestion, reduce overeating, and foster a deeper connection with the food that nourishes you.

As you enjoy your meals, consider:

- **Chewing your food thoroughly:** This aids in digestion and nutrient absorption.
- **Putting your fork down between bites:** This allows you to slow down and savor the flavors.
- **Tuning into your hunger and fullness cues:** Eat

when you're hungry, and stop when you're comfortably satisfied.

- **Noticing how different foods make you feel:** Pay attention to how your body responds to different foods. Do certain foods seem to trigger inflammation or discomfort? Do others make you feel energized and vibrant?

By making mindful choices, one bite at a time, you can nourish your spine, reduce inflammation, and support your body's natural healing abilities. Remember, your plate is a powerful tool for creating a healthier, happier you – from the inside out.

Beyond the Plate: Lifestyle Habits for a Spine-Friendly Life

While nourishing your body with the right nutrients is paramount, a holistic approach to spinal health extends beyond the plate, encompassing the way you move, manage stress, and prioritize rest and recovery.

The Movement Connection: Where Nutrition and Exercise Intertwine

Think about building a house. You wouldn't just lay a solid foundation and call it a day, right? You need the walls, the roof, the whole structure to make it strong and resilient. It's the same with our bodies.

Sure, good nutrition is like that solid foundation, providing the essential building blocks. But without regular exercise, it's like we're missing the framework. Our spines, especially, need movement to stay healthy. It's like giving them a good stretch and workout, strengthening the muscles that support them, keeping them flexible and pain-free.

And here's the magic: when we combine nourishing food with regular movement, it's like a superpower for our bodies. They become incredibly efficient at healing, repairing, and thriving. It's a beautiful synergy that keeps us feeling our best.

Stress Management: Calming the Nervous System, Easing the Pain

Remember those stress hormones, cortisol and adrenaline, we talked about? They're like our body's emergency responders, great in a pinch, but terrible houseguests when they overstay their welcome. When stress becomes a constant companion, these hormones can really start to mess things up. Think inflammation, tight muscles, a grumpy gut, sleepless nights, and even feeling pain more intensely.

It's like our nervous system is a finely tuned instrument, and chronic stress is that one jarring note that keeps getting played, throwing everything off-key.

But here's the good news: we can help our nervous system

find its harmony again. By incorporating stress-reducing practices into our daily lives, we're essentially giving it a soothing massage, allowing it to heal and function at its best.

Here are a few simple yet powerful practices to explore:

- **Deep Breathing:** Even a few minutes of deep, conscious breathing can help calm your nervous system, reduce stress hormones, and alleviate muscle tension.
- **Meditation:** This practice of quieting the mind and cultivating present-moment awareness has been shown to reduce stress, improve sleep, and even decrease pain perception.
- **Yoga:** This ancient practice combines physical postures, breathing exercises, and meditation, promoting flexibility, strength, relaxation, and stress reduction.
- **Nature Immersion:** Spending time in nature has a profoundly calming effect on the nervous system.

Ready to experience the transformative power of food as medicine? We can create a nutrition plan tailored to your specific needs, helping you overcome back or joint pain and reclaim your health from the inside out.

Melody's Lifesavers: From Back Pain to Family Fun

"These ladies are life savers. Earlier this year, they diagnosed my sudden onset of back pain, a dislocated rib, pretty much immediately. I went from nearly immobile to my normal self in no time with their care. My son is also benefiting, and I wish I had taken him in sooner. They hosted us today for a family fun fest too! Everyone in the office is just simply the best."

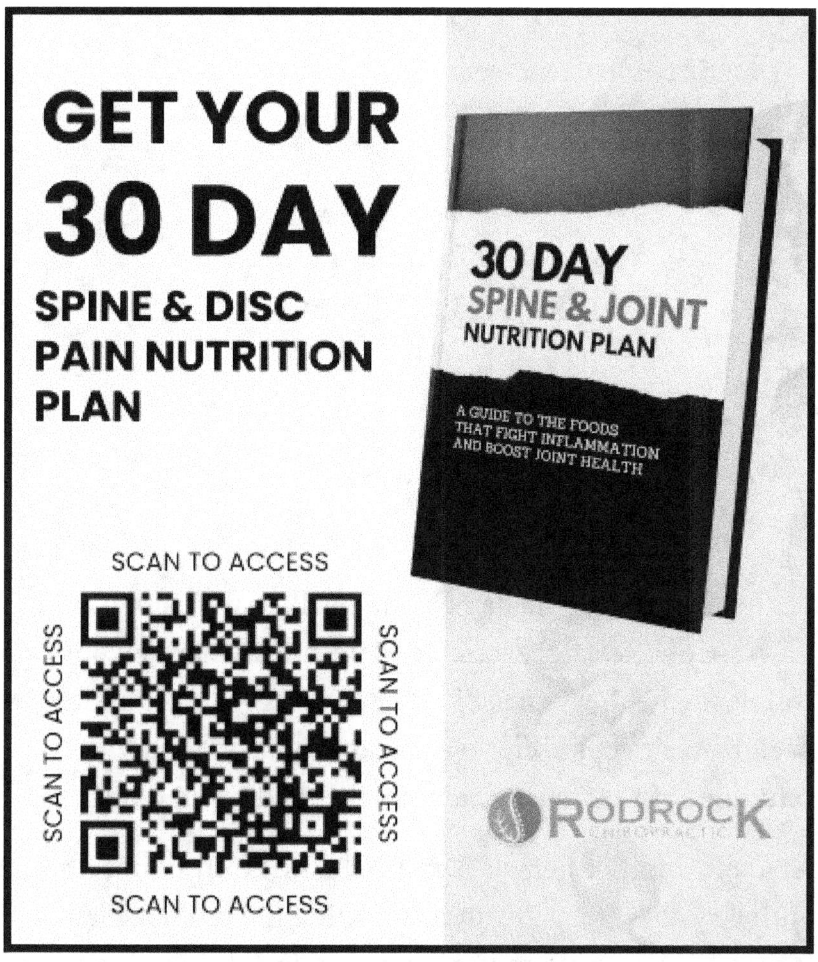

Take back your life from pain. Call 785-465-5605 and discover a natural path to lasting relief.

** Individual results may vary. Please review the disclaimer after the Table of Contents.*

** Results are not typical. Your experience may vary.*

7

THE RESTORE DIFFERENCE

We'll never forget the day Crystal walked into our Lawrence office, her face etched with pain, her newborn son nestled in her arms. She'd been struggling with intense back pain since his birth, each movement a jarring reminder of the invisible enemy that had taken hold.

As a new mother herself, Dr. Amelia instantly connected with Crystal's struggle, understanding the unique challenges of navigating motherhood while battling discomfort. With a gentle touch and a deep understanding of the body's innate healing capacity, Dr. Amelia adjusted Crystal's spine, aiming to restore proper alignment and ease the strain that childbirth can often place on a woman's body.

The results were remarkable. Crystal felt immediate relief, a sense of lightness replacing the persistent ache that had become her constant companion. "I walked in there in pain and, with just one adjustment, was feeling so much better!" she later shared, her words filled with gratitude.

Crystal's experience with the RESTORE Framework is just one example of what's possible, but it's important to note that individual results can vary. What remains consistent is our commitment to providing personalized care and empowering our patients to reclaim their health and well-being.

Crystal's story, like so many others we've witnessed over the years, underscores a powerful truth: the body possesses an incredible capacity for healing, a natural intelligence that, when guided and supported, can lead to profound transformation. This understanding is at the heart of the RESTORE Framework, and it's why we believe in a more nuanced approach to pain relief, one that moves beyond the allure of quick fixes and embraces a deeper, more sustainable path towards healing.

A Foundation Built on Science and Natural Healing

In an era characterized by a constant pursuit of instant gratification, it's easy to be lured by promises of quick pain relief. However, sustainable and meaningful healing often requires a more nuanced approach.

The RESTORE Framework distinguishes itself by grounding its principles in a robust foundation of evidence-based practices. It seamlessly integrates scientific research with time-honored natural healing modalities, recognizing the body's inherent capacity for self-repair.

This chapter will illuminate the scientific underpinnings of the RESTORE Framework, examining the research and guiding principles that enable us to facilitate lasting pain relief and promote overall well-being in our patients.

Beyond Anecdotes: The Importance of Evidence-Based Practices

The RESTORE Framework isn't based on fads, trends, or anecdotal evidence; it's rooted in a commitment to utilizing treatments and therapies that have been rigorously studied and proven effective through scientific research.

We believe in transparency and want you to understand the science behind our approach. We stay abreast of the latest research in pain management, chiropractic care, nutrition, and complementary therapies to ensure that our methods are aligned with the most current scientific understanding.

When evaluating a treatment option, we consider:

- **Scientific Rigor:** Is the treatment supported by well-designed studies published in reputable medical journals?
- **Clinical Trials:** Has the treatment been tested in

controlled clinical trials involving a significant number of participants?

- **Safety and Efficacy:** Does the research demonstrate both the safety and effectiveness of the treatment?
- **Long-Term Outcomes:** Does the treatment provide lasting relief, or are the benefits merely temporary?

Our commitment to evidence-based practices ensures that you receive the highest quality care, backed by scientific rigor and a dedication to achieving optimal outcomes.

The Power Within: Harnessing the Efficacy of Natural Remedies

The human body is a marvel of nature—a self-healing, self-regulating organism with an innate capacity to repair and regenerate. The RESTORE Framework honors this innate wisdom, incorporating natural remedies and therapies that work in harmony with your body's inherent healing abilities.

These natural approaches offer a gentle yet powerful alternative to conventional pain management, often providing relief without the risk of harsh side effects or dependence associated with some medications.

We incorporate a variety of natural remedies, including:

- **Chiropractic Adjustments:** These gentle, precise adjustments to the spine help restore proper joint alignment, reduce nerve interference, and optimize nervous system function—all crucial for promoting natural healing.
- **Acupuncture:** This ancient practice utilizes strategically placed, ultra-thin needles to stimulate specific points along the body's energy meridians, promoting pain relief, reducing inflammation, and restoring balance.
- **Nutritional Therapy:** We believe that food is medicine and can provide personalized guidance on dietary choices that nourish your spine, reduce inflammation, and support your body's natural healing processes.

These natural remedies, often used in conjunction with other evidence-based therapies, form a powerful synergy that addresses the root cause of your pain and empowers your body to heal from within.

Unlocking Your Inner Healer: The Body's Astonishing Capacity for Self-Repair

The human body is a marvel of biological engineering, capable of astonishing feats of self-repair and regeneration. At every moment, complex processes are underway—cellular repair, tissue reconstruction, wound closure—all driven by an intricate network of systems working in concert.

The RESTORE Framework recognizes and respects this inherent healing capacity. We understand that true, sustainable relief stems not from simply suppressing symptoms, but from fostering an environment conducive to the body's natural healing processes.

Consider the body's own internal regulatory mechanisms as a highly sophisticated physician, constantly monitoring and adjusting functions to maintain optimal health. Pain or injury often signals that this internal physician is encountering interference, that something is impeding its ability to function effectively.

The RESTORE approach focuses on identifying and addressing these impediments—be they structural misalignments, muscular imbalances, nutritional deficiencies, or chronic stress responses. By removing these obstacles, we empower the body's innate healing mechanisms to restore balance and well-being.

This means:

- **Restoring Proper Alignment:** Chiropractic adjustments address misalignments in the spine that can interfere with nerve function, muscle balance, and overall biomechanics.

- **Releasing Tension and Restrictions:** Massage therapy helps to release muscle tension, improve circulation, and reduce inflammation, allowing tissues to heal more effectively.
- **Balancing Energy Flow:** Acupuncture helps to restore the flow of vital energy (Qi) throughout the body, promoting pain relief, reducing inflammation, and supporting overall balance.
- **Nourishing from Within:** Nutrition plays a vital role in providing the building blocks your body needs for repair and regeneration.
- **Calming the Nervous System:** Stress management techniques help to reduce the impact of stress hormones on your body, creating an environment that is conducive to healing.

By working *with* your body's innate healing wisdom, rather than against it, the RESTORE Framework empowers you to experience lasting relief, reclaim your vitality, and unlock your full potential for health and well-being.

Beyond the Conventional: Embracing the Holistic Healthcare Revolution

For years, we've relied on a medical system that's like a skilled mechanic, brilliant at fixing broken parts and patching up emergencies. It's saved countless lives and given us incredible tools to combat acute illnesses. But what happens when the problem isn't a broken bone or a sudden infection? What about the persistent aches, the nagging fatigue, the invisible struggles that define chronic conditions?

There's a growing sense that we need something more, a healthcare approach that sees us as whole beings, not just a collection of symptoms. It's about recognizing the intricate dance between our physical health, our mental well-being, and even our sense of purpose. This shift towards a more holistic view is gaining momentum, promising a future where healthcare truly nourishes the whole person.

A New Perspective: Embracing a Paradigm Shift in Healthcare

The holistic healthcare revolution represents a fundamental shift in perspective. It's a move away from viewing the body as a collection of isolated parts and towards recognizing it as a complex, interconnected system where every element influences the others.

This paradigm shift involves:

- **Addressing the Root Cause:** Rather than simply masking symptoms, holistic healthcare seeks to uncover and address the underlying causes of illness and pain.
- **Empowering Patients:** Patients are no longer passive recipients of care; they become active participants in their healing journey, making informed decisions and taking ownership of their health.
- **Integrating Multiple Modalities:** Holistic healthcare embraces a wide range of treatment options, blending conventional medicine with complementary therapies to create a personalized approach tailored to each individual's unique needs.
- **Focusing on Prevention:** Rather than waiting for illness to strike, holistic healthcare emphasizes preventive measures, lifestyle modifications, and strategies to maintain optimal well-being.

A Vision of Wellness: Shaping the Future of Healthcare

The future of healthcare is moving towards a more integrated, holistic model that empowers individuals to take control of their well-being. This exciting evolution involves:

- **Personalized Medicine:** Treatments and therapies will be increasingly tailored to each individual's unique genetic makeup, lifestyle, and health history.
- **Mind-Body Connection:** The profound connection between mental and emotional well-being and physical health will be increasingly recognized and integrated into treatment plans.
- **Technology as a Tool, Not a Replacement:** Technology will continue to advance, providing valuable tools for diagnosis, treatment, and monitoring, but it will be used in conjunction with human touch, compassion, and personalized care.
- **Focus on Lifestyle as Medicine:** The power of lifestyle choices – nutrition, exercise, stress management, and sleep – will be increasingly emphasized as a cornerstone of health and well-being.

The RESTORE Framework is at the forefront of this holistic healthcare revolution. We believe in empowering our patients with knowledge, providing personalized care that addresses the root cause of their pain, and integrating a wide range of therapies to support their journey towards lasting relief and optimal well-being.

Pioneers of Wellness: Leading the Charge for a Holistic Future

At Rodrock Chiropractic, we're not just practitioners; we're passionate advocates for a shift in healthcare – a move away from the limitations of the conventional model and towards a more holistic, patient-centered approach.

We're committed to leading the change by:

- **Providing a Model of Integrated Care:** We blend the best of chiropractic care, massage therapy, acupuncture, and other natural healing modalities with the latest advancements in pain management technology to create a truly comprehensive approach.
- **Empowering Patients Through Education:** We believe that informed patients are empowered patients. We take the time to educate our patients about their conditions, the science behind our approach, and the power of lifestyle choices to support their healing journey.
- **Creating a Community of Wellness:** We foster a supportive, welcoming environment where patients feel heard, respected, and empowered to take ownership of their health.

Driven by Purpose: Our Mission and Values

Our practice is driven by a deep sense of purpose, guiding everything we do, from the way we interact with our patients to the treatments we provide.

Our Mission: Rodrock Chiropractic has an expert health team that specializes in identifying the root cause of your suffering. Our mission is to find the fastest path to healing and restore your body to its optimal function so you are not just surviving in life but thriving.

Our Purpose: To serve every child, woman, and man who walks through our doors with integrity, compassion, and love. We are dedicated to:

- **Finding and Removing Vertebral Subluxations:** Subluxations are misalignments in the spine that can interfere with nerve function and overall well-being. Chiropractic adjustments gently and effectively address these subluxations, allowing the body's innate intelligence to express itself to its optimal potential.
- **Educating Every Patient:** We believe that knowledge is power. We take the time to educate our patients about the true nature of health, the importance of spinal health, and the power they have to take control of their well-being.
- **Creating a Ripple Effect:** We envision a world where holistic healthcare is the norm, where people understand the interconnectedness of their bodies, minds, and spirits, and where everyone has the opportunity to experience a life filled with vitality, joy, and freedom from pain.

The RESTORE Framework isn't just a collection of treatments; it's a philosophy, a commitment to honoring your body's innate healing wisdom and empowering you to reclaim your health. We believe in the power of science, the efficacy of natural remedies, and the transformative potential of a holistic approach.

Are you ready to experience the RESTORE difference? Visit our website, contact our Lawrence or Baldwin City office at 785-465-5605, or simply scan the code below to get in touch with us today. Your journey towards a pain-free, vibrant life starts now. Please note that individual results can vary and are not guaranteed.

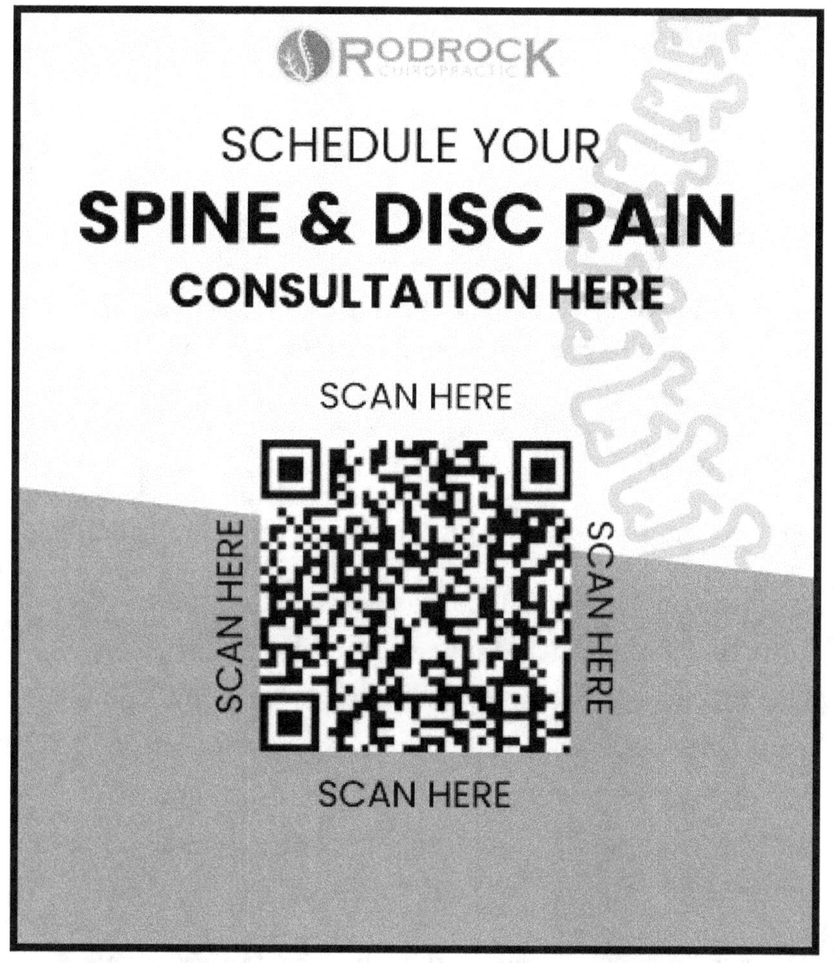

Imagine a life without limitations. Call 785-465-5605 today and let us help you get there.

** Individual results may vary. Please review the disclaimer after the Table of Contents.*

8

ADVANCED HEALING TECHNOLOGIES IN THE RESTORE PROGRAM

The look on Michael's face was one we knew all too well –
a mix of exhaustion and quiet desperation. He'd been
battling chronic back pain for years, cycling through a
seemingly endless carousel of treatments that offered only
fleeting moments of relief. The pain had become a
constant companion, dictating his every move, stealing his
energy, and chipping away at his hope.

"I'm tired of just managing the pain," he confessed, his
voice heavy with frustration. "I want to get back to living
my life."

We understood his yearning, having witnessed the toll that
chronic pain takes on countless individuals. As we guided
Michael through the RESTORE Framework, introducing
him to a holistic approach that addressed not only the

physical symptoms but also the underlying causes of his discomfort, we could see a glimmer of hope rekindled in his eyes.

But there was one particular moment in Michael's journey that truly stands out. It was the day he experienced the Back on Trac Table for the first time. As he lay on the specialized table, feeling the gentle decompression and stretching movements, a wave of relaxation washed over him. For the first time in years, he felt a release of tension, a sense of space opening up between his vertebrae.

"It's like my spine can finally breathe," he remarked, a smile spreading across his face. "I haven't felt this good in years!" While Michael's experience with the Back on Trac Table was incredibly positive, it's important to remember that individual results can vary.

Michael's story highlights a key aspect of the RESTORE Framework: we believe in integrating cutting-edge technologies with traditional healing modalities to accelerate the body's natural healing process. These advanced healing technologies aren't magic bullets; they are powerful tools that, when used strategically within a holistic framework, can empower individuals to achieve profound and lasting relief.

Back on Trac Table: Relieving Spinal Pressure and Restoring Alignment

Have you ever wished for a magic wand to erase the aches and pains that seem to weigh you down? The Back on Trac table might be the closest thing we have. Imagine sinking into this specialized chair and feeling a gentle, almost weightless sensation as it gently lifts the pressure from your spine. It's like a sigh of relief for your entire body.

This isn't magic, though. It's science. The Back on Trac table uses a clever combination of gentle stretching and controlled movements to create space between your vertebrae. Think of it as giving your spine a little breathing room, allowing those compressed discs and nerves to finally relax. This decompression can be particularly beneficial for individuals experiencing:

- **Chronic back pain:** By alleviating pressure on irritated nerves, the Back on Trac table can provide significant relief from nagging back pain.
- **Sciatica:** This condition, characterized by pain radiating down the leg, often stems from a compressed sciatic nerve. Spinal decompression can help free the nerve, reducing pain and improving mobility.
- **Herniated discs:** When the soft, jelly-like center of a spinal disc pushes through its outer layer, it can cause pain and inflammation. The Back on Trac

table can help reposition the disc, reducing pressure and promoting healing.

Beyond pain relief, the Back on Trac table also promotes spinal alignment and improved posture. By gently stretching and mobilizing the spine, it helps restore its natural curvature and encourages proper alignment. This can lead to:

- **Increased flexibility and range of motion:** As spinal restrictions are released, individuals often experience greater ease of movement and flexibility.
- **Improved posture:** By addressing spinal misalignments, the Back on Trac table can help individuals stand taller and maintain a more balanced posture.
- **Reduced muscle tension:** When the spine is properly aligned, muscles are less likely to become strained or tense, leading to overall relaxation and reduced pain.

The Back on Trac table is a non-invasive, drug-free approach to spinal health that complements other therapies within the RESTORE program. It's a powerful tool for restoring spinal integrity, relieving pain, and empowering individuals to move with greater ease and confidence.

SoftWave Therapy: Accelerating Healing from Within

What if the key to unlocking your body's healing potential lies not in drugs or surgery, but in sound? SoftWave Therapy delves into the fascinating world of acoustic medicine, using precisely calibrated sound waves to awaken dormant healing powers within.

Imagine these waves as tiny messengers, traveling deep into your tissues, gently coaxing cells back to life and igniting a chain reaction of repair. It's a revolutionary approach that's changing the way we think about pain and recovery.

Here's how SoftWave Therapy works its magic:

- **Reduces Inflammation:** The acoustic waves effectively target inflamed tissues, reducing swelling and pain. This is particularly beneficial for conditions like arthritis, tendinitis, and muscle strains.
- **Promotes Healing:** By stimulating blood flow and nutrient delivery to injured areas, SoftWave Therapy accelerates the healing process. This can significantly shorten recovery times for a wide range of musculoskeletal injuries.
- **Activates Stem Cell Regeneration:** One of the most exciting aspects of SoftWave Therapy is its

ability to stimulate stem cell activity. Stem cells are the body's master repair cells, capable of differentiating into various cell types and contributing to tissue regeneration. By activating these cells, SoftWave Therapy can enhance the body's natural ability to heal and repair itself.

Cutting Healing Time in Half:

While individual results may vary, many patients experience a dramatic reduction in healing time with SoftWave Therapy. By addressing the root cause of pain and inflammation and promoting optimal healing conditions, SoftWave Therapy can help individuals get back to their active lives faster and with less discomfort.

Beyond Pain Relief:

SoftWave Therapy isn't just for acute injuries. It can also be used to address chronic pain conditions, improve mobility, and enhance overall tissue health.

A Holistic Approach to Healing:

SoftWave Therapy is a powerful tool that complements other therapies within the RESTORE program. By combining this cutting-edge technology with personalized treatment plans, we empower individuals to achieve optimal healing and well-being.

Red Light Therapy: Bathing Your Body in Healing Light

Have you ever imagined a therapy that could soothe your aches and pains with the gentle warmth of light? That's the promise of Red Light Therapy, a fascinating, drug-free approach that's making waves in the wellness world.

Picture this: specific wavelengths of red and near-infrared light, like tiny beams of sunshine, penetrating deep into your tissues. It's like giving your cells a revitalizing bath, sparking a chain reaction of healing and rejuvenation at the most fundamental level.

Turning Down the Inflammatory Fire:

One of the key benefits of Red Light Therapy is its ability to reduce inflammation. When tissues are injured or inflamed, the body releases inflammatory molecules that can cause pain, swelling, and stiffness. Red light therapy helps to modulate this inflammatory response, calming the "fire" and promoting a more balanced healing environment.

How Does It Work?

Red light therapy works by stimulating mitochondria, the powerhouses of our cells. These tiny organelles are responsible for producing energy (ATP) that fuels cellular processes. By boosting mitochondrial function, red light therapy enhances cellular energy production, which in turn supports:

- **Reduced inflammation:** Increased energy production allows cells to better regulate inflammatory responses.
- **Accelerated healing:** Enhanced cellular function promotes tissue repair and regeneration.
- **Pain relief:** By reducing inflammation and improving circulation, red light therapy can alleviate pain.

Beyond Inflammation:

Red Light Therapy offers a wide range of potential benefits beyond reducing inflammation, including:

- **Improved skin health:** Red light therapy can stimulate collagen production, reduce wrinkles, and improve skin tone.
- **Enhanced muscle recovery:** It can help reduce muscle soreness and accelerate recovery after exercise.
- **Improved sleep quality:** Red light therapy can help regulate circadian rhythms and promote restful sleep.

A Gentle and Effective Therapy:

Red Light Therapy is a safe, non-invasive, and painless therapy that can be used to address a variety of health concerns. It's a powerful tool that complements other therapies within the RESTORE program, helping individuals achieve optimal well-being.

The technologies explored in this chapter represent more than just isolated treatments; they are integral components of the RESTORE program's holistic philosophy. By addressing the interconnectedness of body, mind, and spirit, these tools work in synergy to create a comprehensive healing experience.

As you progress through the program, you'll discover how this integrated approach fosters not only physical recovery but also a profound sense of well-being.

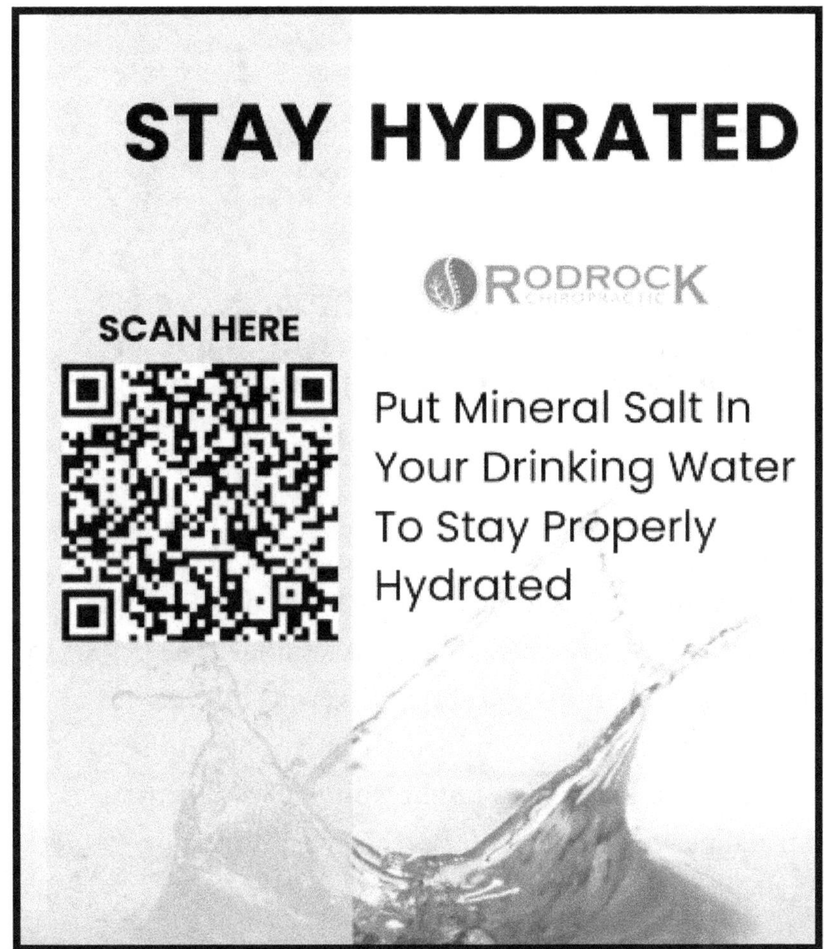

You deserve to live pain-free. Call 785-465-5605 and take the first step towards a healthier, happier you.

** Individual results may vary. Please review the disclaimer after the Table of Contents.*

9

THE POSTURE PRESCRIPTION: YOUR GUIDE TO ALIGNING YOUR BODY FOR OPTIMAL HEALTH AND WELL-BEING

Imagine this: you're hunched over your computer, engrossed in your work, when that familiar ache begins to creep into your neck and shoulders. You shift in your chair, trying to find a comfortable position, but the discomfort persists. You might wonder, "Is this just a normal part of modern life? Is this what it feels like to get older?"

We're here to tell you that you don't have to accept pain and discomfort as inevitable consequences of a desk job, technology use, or simply living in a modern world. By understanding the power of posture and ergonomics – the science of designing your environment to fit your body – you can transform your comfort, prevent pain, and reclaim your mobility.

Good posture isn't about standing rigidly straight or forcing yourself into unnatural positions. It's about creating a supportive environment for your body, allowing your spine to function optimally, and minimizing stress on your joints and muscles. It's about moving with ease, grace, and a sense of freedom.

Posture Principles: Finding Your Natural Alignment

Good posture isn't about achieving a rigid, picture-perfect stance; it's about finding a natural, balanced alignment that minimizes stress on your body and allows you to move with ease and grace.

Here are the basic principles of proper posture:

- **Head Balanced Over Shoulders:** Imagine a string gently pulling the crown of your head towards the sky. Your ears should be aligned with your shoulders, and your chin should be slightly tucked. Avoid jutting your head forward, which can strain your neck muscles.
- **Shoulders Over Hips:** Your shoulders should be relaxed and slightly pulled back, aligning with your hips. Avoid rounding your shoulders forward, which can lead to tightness in your chest and weakness in your upper back muscles.
- **Natural Spinal Curves Maintained:** Your spine has natural curves – a slight inward curve in your

lower back (lordosis), an outward curve in your upper back (kyphosis), and a slight inward curve in your neck (cervical lordosis). Maintaining these curves is essential for shock absorption, flexibility, and optimal spinal health.

Debunking Posture Myths:

- **Myth:** You need to stand perfectly straight, like a soldier at attention.
- **Reality:** While standing tall is important, forcing yourself into an overly rigid posture can be uncomfortable and unsustainable. Focus on finding a natural alignment that feels balanced and relaxed.
- **Myth:** Slouching is always bad.
- **Reality:** While prolonged slouching can lead to muscle imbalances and pain, our bodies are designed for movement and flexibility. It's perfectly normal and healthy to shift positions throughout the day. The key is to avoid staying in any one position for too long.
- **Myth:** Good posture is only about appearances.
- **Reality:** While good posture can make you look taller and more confident, its benefits go far beyond aesthetics. Proper alignment supports optimal spinal health, reduces strain on joints and

muscles, improves breathing, and can even boost energy levels.

- **Myth:** Once you have bad posture, you're stuck with it.
- **Reality:** While it takes time and effort to improve posture, it's never too late to make changes. With consistent awareness, targeted exercises, and ergonomic adjustments, you can retrain your muscles, improve your alignment, and experience the benefits of better posture.
- **Myth:** Only people with back pain need to worry about posture.
- **Reality:** Everyone can benefit from good posture. It's essential for preventing pain and injury, maintaining mobility as you age, and supporting overall health and well-being.

Good posture isn't about achieving perfection or conforming to a rigid ideal. It's about finding what feels natural, balanced, and comfortable for your body.

Simple Posture Checks:

- **Standing:**
- **Wall Test:** Stand with your back flat against a wall, heels a few inches away. Your head, shoulders, and buttocks should touch the wall, with a small space between your lower back and the wall.

- **Earlobe Over Shoulder, Shoulder Over Hip:** Imagine a plumb line dropping from your earlobe through your shoulder and down to your hip. These points should be aligned.
- **Tall and Proud Feeling:** When your posture is aligned, you should feel a sense of being tall, balanced, and energized.
- **Sitting:**
- **Feet Flat on the Floor:** Your feet should be flat on the floor, with your knees slightly lower than your hips. If your feet don't reach the floor, use a footrest.
- **Chair Back Supporting Lower Back:** Choose a chair with good lumbar support that fits the natural curve of your lower back.
- **Computer Screen at Eye Level:** Position your computer monitor so the top of the screen is at eye level. This will help prevent you from hunching over your work.

By incorporating these simple posture checks into your daily routine, you can become more aware of your alignment and make adjustments to promote a healthier, more comfortable posture.

Taming the Desk Job Beast: Ergonomics for a Pain-Free Workday

The sedentary nature of many modern jobs presents a significant challenge to musculoskeletal health. Prolonged sitting, coupled with repetitive movements and poor posture, can contribute to a range of issues, from minor aches and pains to chronic conditions.

Fortunately, the field of ergonomics offers evidence-based solutions to mitigate these risks. By applying ergonomic principles to the design and arrangement of the work-space, individuals can significantly reduce their risk of developing work-related musculoskeletal disorders. This involves optimizing factors such as chair height, desk surface level, monitor placement, and keyboard ergonomics to promote neutral postures and minimize strain on the body.

Workspace Makeover: Creating an Ergonomic Oasis

Think of your workspace as an extension of your body, a space that should support your natural alignment and minimize strain on your muscles and joints. Here are some key adjustments to consider:

- **The Throne of Comfort: Your Chair:**
- **Adjustability is Key:** Invest in a chair with adjustable height, lumbar support, and armrests.

Your feet should be flat on the floor, with your knees slightly lower than your hips.

- **Lumbar Support:** Ensure the chair provides adequate support for the natural curve of your lower back. Use a lumbar support cushion if needed.
- **Armrest Alignment:** Adjust the armrests so your shoulders are relaxed, and your elbows are bent at a 90-degree angle.
- **Desk Dynamics: Standing Tall**
- **Proper Height:** Your desk should be at a height that allows you to work comfortably with your elbows bent at a 90-degree angle and your wrists straight.
- **Standing Desk Option:** Consider a standing desk or a desk converter that allows you to alternate between sitting and standing throughout the day.
- **Monitor Magic: Eye-to-Screen Harmony**
- **Position:** Your monitor should be positioned directly in front of you, with the top of the screen at eye level.
- **Distance:** Maintain a comfortable distance from the screen—about an arm's length away.
- **Keyboard and Mouse Mastery: Wrist-Friendly Zones**
- **Proximity:** Your keyboard and mouse should be close enough to avoid reaching and straining your shoulders.

- **Wrist Alignment:** Keep your wrists straight while typing and using the mouse.
- **Support:** Use a mouse pad with wrist support to minimize pressure on your wrist joints.

Beyond the Chair: The Power of Movement Breaks

You know how they say "sitting is the new smoking"? Well, there's some truth to it! Even if your desk setup is ergonomic heaven, spending hours glued to your chair isn't doing your body any favors. We humans are built to move, and staying put for too long can leave you feeling stiff, achy, and sluggish.

But don't worry, there's a simple fix: movement breaks! Think of them as mini-vacations for your body. Every hour, get up and stretch those legs, take a quick stroll around the office, or just stand up and shake things up. These little bursts of activity can work wonders for your comfort and prevent the sneaky build-up of tension from all that sitting.

Ergonomics Beyond the Desk: Posture Power-Ups for Everyday Life

Ergonomics isn't just for the office; it's a mindset, a way of approaching everyday activities with an awareness of how your body moves and interacts with its surroundings. By applying ergonomic principles to your daily life, you can minimize strain, prevent pain, and protect your spine and joints for years to come.

Mindful Movement: Ergonomics for Everyday Activities

We often perform everyday tasks on autopilot, barely thinking about how we move. But bringing awareness to these seemingly simple actions can make a world of difference in preventing pain and injury.

Here are a few tips for incorporating ergonomics into your daily routines:

- **Lifting Like a Pro:**
- **Bend at the Knees:** When lifting heavy objects, always bend at your knees, keeping your back straight. Use your leg muscles, not your back, to lift.
- **Avoid Twisting:** Never twist while lifting. Turn your whole body instead.
- **Keep It Close:** Hold the object close to your body to minimize strain on your back.
- **Carrying with Ease:**
- **Distribute Weight Evenly:** When carrying bags or groceries, distribute the weight evenly on both sides of your body.
- **Backpack Power:** Use a backpack instead of a shoulder bag to distribute weight more evenly and prevent strain on one shoulder.
- **Lighten the Load:** Avoid carrying excessively

heavy loads. Break down large loads into smaller, more manageable ones.

- **Driving in Comfort:**
- **Seat Adjustment:** Adjust your seat so you can easily reach the pedals and steering wheel while maintaining a comfortable posture. Your knees should be slightly bent, and your back should be supported.
- **Lumbar Support:** Use a lumbar support cushion if your car seat doesn't provide adequate support for your lower back.
- **Take Breaks:** On long drives, take frequent breaks to stretch and move around.

Taming Tech Neck: Saving Your Neck From the Digital Age

We love our smartphones and tablets, but all that screen time comes at a price – tech neck. Hours spent staring down at devices can strain our neck muscles, leading to pain, stiffness, headaches, and even long-term postural problems.

Here's how to protect your neck in the digital age:

- **Elevate Your Devices:** Hold your phone or tablet at eye level, rather than hunching over it.
- **Take Frequent Breaks:** Every 20-30 minutes, look away from your screen, stretch your neck, and

focus on a distant object to give your eye muscles a break.

- **Strengthen Your Neck Muscles:** Incorporate neck stretches and exercises into your routine to strengthen the muscles that support your head and neck.

By bringing awareness to your posture and movements throughout the day – at work, at home, and everywhere in between – you can create a more supportive environment for your body, minimize pain, and prevent long-term damage.

Beyond Mechanics: The Mind-Body Connection and the Power of Awareness

Improving your posture isn't just about making external adjustments to your workspace or remembering the "correct" way to stand and sit. It's also about cultivating a deeper awareness of your body – tuning into its subtle signals, noticing habits that contribute to pain, and making mindful choices throughout the day.

Posture Check-Ins: Becoming a Posture Detective

In our busy lives, we often move through our days on autopilot, barely noticing how we're holding our bodies. But bringing conscious awareness to your posture is the first step towards making lasting changes.

Think of it like this: imagine you're driving a car, but you only glance at the road occasionally. You might miss important signs, make wrong turns, or even end up in a ditch. Similarly, if you're not paying attention to your posture, you might be unknowingly straining your muscles, stressing your joints, and setting yourself up for pain.

The Power of Micro-Adjustments:

Making small, consistent adjustments throughout the day is far more effective than trying to force yourself into perfect posture for short periods. Think of it like steering a ship – a small adjustment to the rudder can significantly alter the ship's course over time.

Here's how to incorporate posture check-ins into your day:

- **Set Reminders:** Use your phone, computer, or watch to set reminders to check your posture throughout the day.
- **Use Visual Cues:** Place sticky notes on your computer monitor, mirror, or refrigerator to remind you to stand tall or adjust your alignment.
- **Link to Existing Habits:** Connect your posture check-ins to habits you already do regularly, such as getting up to refill your water bottle, taking a bathroom break, or answering the phone.

Gentle Corrections: The Power of Consistency

Forget about aiming for picture-perfect posture – that's a recipe for frustration! Instead, think of it as a gentle journey of rediscovering your body's natural alignment.

Notice yourself slumping? Shoulders creeping up towards your ears? Take a moment to gently coax yourself back into a more upright position. It's like whispering a reminder to your muscles, "Hey, remember how good it feels to stand tall?"

The secret sauce? Consistency. Those little tweaks you make throughout the day, like tiny seeds of change, will slowly blossom into a more balanced and comfortable posture. It's about listening to your body, honoring its whispers, and creating a foundation for movement that feels as effortless as a summer breeze.

Stand Tall, Live Well: Embracing a Posture-Empowered Life

The RESTORE Framework empowers you to take an active role in your well-being, recognizing that true health is a journey, not a destination. And good posture is an integral part of that journey—a proactive choice you make every day to support your spine, prevent pain, and enhance your overall vitality.

Achieving optimal posture isn't about attaining a rigid, picture-perfect stance. It's about finding a natural alignment that feels balanced and comfortable for *your* body. It's about moving with ease, grace, and a sense of freedom.

It's about making mindful choices throughout your day—adjusting your workspace, incorporating movement breaks, being aware of how you sit, stand, and lift, and even paying attention to how you hold your phone.

It's about cultivating a deeper connection with your body, tuning into its signals, and making adjustments that support its natural alignment.

And it's about remembering that good posture is an ongoing practice, not a destination. There will be days when you slouch, moments when you forget to adjust your workspace, and times when old habits creep back in. That's okay. The key is to gently correct your course, to keep practicing, and to celebrate every step you take towards a more balanced, comfortable, and pain-free life.

Ready to unlock your posture potential and experience the transformative power of proper alignment? Click here to contact us at Rodrock Chiropractic today. We offer personalized postural assessments, gentle chiropractic adjustments, and ergonomic guidance to help you stand tall, move with ease, and live well.

ACTION STEP: Get Your Spine and Joint Pain Relief Handbook. Master 11 Key Stretches from Home To

Retrain Your Spine and Restore Your Discs.

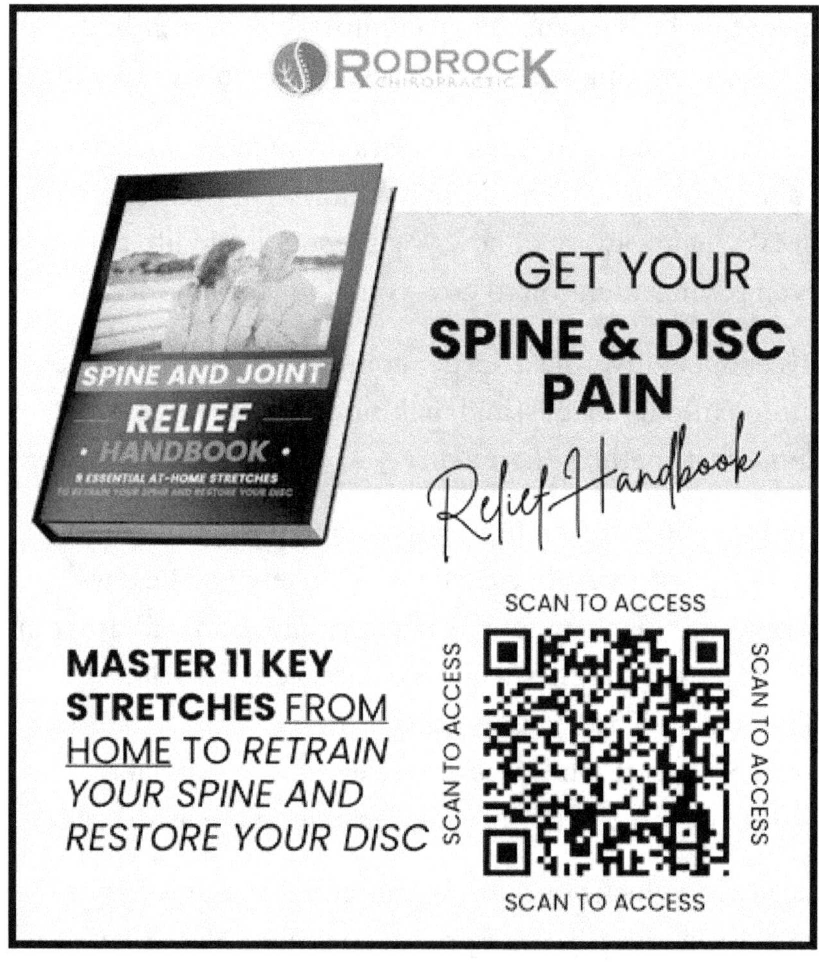

Keith's 5-Star Review: Rodrock Chiropractic is the Best for Back, Neck & Concussion Issues

Dr. Jeremy and his staff are not only friendly and professional, they're unbelievable! The environment is amazing, and Jeremy really knows what he's doing. I'd recommend him to anyone for back, neck, concussion issues, or even a simple sports physical. Hands down, he's the best!

Unlock your body's natural healing power. Call 785-465-5605 and experience the RESTORE difference.

** Individual results may vary. Please review the disclaimer after the Table of Contents.*

** This is one individual's experience and does not guarantee similar results.*

10

PAIN RELIEF FROM WITHIN: HOW TO HARNESS YOUR MIND TO MANAGE DISCOMFORT AND RECLAIM YOUR LIFE

Chronic pain is more than just a physical sensation; it's a complex experience that can profoundly impact mental health. Imagine being constantly bombarded by a relentless wave of discomfort, a feeling that permeates every aspect of your life. This chapter sheds light on the often-overlooked connection between chronic pain and mental well-being.

We'll delve into how pain can influence our thoughts, emotions, and overall sense of self. From anxiety and depression to social isolation and sleep disturbances, the ripple effects of chronic pain can be far-reaching. But there is hope. This chapter equips you with knowledge and practical strategies to manage pain's physical and emotional dimensions, empowering you to reclaim your life and find a path toward holistic healing.

Beyond the Physical: Recognizing the Complexity of Pain

For far too long, pain has been treated as a purely physical phenomenon, a signal that something is broken or damaged in the body. But anyone who has experienced chronic pain knows that it goes far deeper than just aching muscles or stiff joints. Pain is a complex experience, a symphony of sensations, emotions, thoughts, and beliefs intertwined within the intricate tapestry of our nervous system.

Imagine this: two people experience the same injury – a sprained ankle, for example. One person might feel a sharp, intense pain initially, but as the injury heals, their pain gradually subsides, and they're able to resume their normal activities relatively quickly. The other person, however, might experience persistent pain that lingers long after the tissues have healed, affecting their mood, their sleep, their relationships, and their overall quality of life.

What accounts for this difference? Why do some people experience pain more intensely or for longer durations than others?

The answer lies in the complex interplay between the physical sensation of pain and our thoughts, emotions, and beliefs about pain. Chronic pain can trigger a cascade of psychological and emotional responses:

- **Fear of Movement:** You might become afraid to move, fearing that any activity will worsen your pain, leading to decreased activity, muscle weakness, and a vicious cycle of pain and immobility.
- **Anxiety and Depression:** Living with constant pain can be emotionally draining, leading to feelings of anxiety, helplessness, hopelessness, and even depression.
- **Social Isolation:** Pain can make it difficult to participate in social activities, leading to withdrawal from friends and family and a sense of isolation.
- **Negative Thoughts and Beliefs:** You might develop negative thoughts and beliefs about your pain, such as "I'll never get better," "This pain will control my life," or "I'm a burden to others."

These emotional and psychological responses can, in turn, amplify your perception of pain, making it feel more intense and harder to manage. This complex interplay highlights the need for a holistic approach to pain management – one that addresses both the physical *and* the emotional aspects of this multifaceted experience.

The Pain-Emotion Cycle: A Two-Way Street

Chronic pain and mental health are intricately inter-twined, influencing each other in a complex, bidirectional dance. It's not simply a one-way street where pain causes emotional distress; mental health struggles can also worsen pain perception, making it harder to cope and recover.

Imagine two gears, tightly interlocked. When one gear turns, it inevitably sets the other in motion. Similarly, chronic pain and emotional well-being are constantly influencing each other, creating a cycle that can be difficult to break.

Here's how this two-way street unfolds:

- **Pain Fuels Emotional Distress:** Living with persistent pain can take a toll on your emotional well-being. The constant discomfort, the limitations it imposes on your life, and the uncertainty about the future can trigger feelings of frustration, anxiety, sadness, and even hopelessness.
- **Emotional Distress Amplifies Pain:** Conversely, when you're struggling with anxiety, depression, or other mental health challenges, your perception of pain can intensify. Stress hormones, released during times of emotional distress, can heighten

your sensitivity to pain signals, making even minor aches and discomfort feel more intense.

This cyclical relationship between pain and emotional well-being can create a downward spiral, making it increasingly difficult to manage both your physical and mental health.

Common Mental Health Challenges Faced by Those with Chronic Pain

It's essential to recognize that experiencing emotional distress alongside chronic pain is not a sign of weakness. These struggles are real, valid, and often a natural response to the challenges of living with persistent discomfort.

Here are some of the most common mental health challenges faced by individuals with chronic pain:

- **Depression:** Persistent pain can lead to feelings of hopelessness, loss of interest in activities you once enjoyed, changes in sleep and appetite, fatigue, difficulty concentrating, and social withdrawal.
- **Anxiety:** Chronic pain can trigger constant worry about the pain, fear of movement or re-injury, panic attacks, and a heightened sense of vigilance and tension in the body.
- **Sleep Disorders:** Pain can disrupt sleep, making it difficult to fall asleep, stay asleep, or achieve restful sleep. This sleep deprivation, in turn, can worsen

pain, fatigue, mood, and cognitive function, creating a vicious cycle.

If you're experiencing any of these challenges, know that you're not alone. Seeking support from a qualified mental health professional, alongside addressing the physical aspects of your pain, is essential for breaking free from this cycle and reclaiming your overall well-being.

You are not weak or flawed for struggling emotionally when you're in pain. Your experience is valid, and there are effective strategies and compassionate support available to help you navigate this challenging journey.

CBT: Rewiring Your Relationship with Pain

Chronic pain can be a relentless storm, battering your mind and body. While medication and physical therapy offer shelter, Cognitive Behavioral Therapy (CBT) provides the compass and map to navigate the tempest. It's a powerful, evidence-based approach that recognizes the intricate dance between our thoughts, feelings, and behaviors.

Imagine your pain as a raging river. Traditional treatments might build dams to contain the water, but CBT teaches you to build bridges. It equips you with the skills to cross the river, to find new paths and perspectives, ultimately lessening the river's power over your life. CBT doesn't erase the pain, but it empowers you to live alongside it, to find peace and purpose even in the midst of the storm.

The Core Principles of CBT

CBT is based on the understanding that our thoughts, feelings, and behaviors are interconnected and influence each other. By changing negative thought patterns and developing healthy coping mechanisms, you can reduce emotional distress, improve your ability to manage pain, and ultimately reclaim a sense of control over your life.

Here are the core principles of CBT for pain management:

- **Identifying and Challenging Negative Thoughts:** CBT helps you become aware of automatic negative thoughts that can amplify pain perception and make it harder to cope. For example, if you're experiencing a pain flare-up, you might automatically think, "This is never going to end," or "I'm going to be stuck in pain forever." CBT helps you recognize these thoughts, challenge their validity, and replace them with more balanced and realistic perspectives.
- **Developing Effective Coping Strategies:** CBT provides you with a toolbox of practical coping strategies to manage pain flare-ups, reduce anxiety, and improve your overall mood. These strategies might include relaxation techniques (deep breathing, progressive muscle relaxation),

mindfulness exercises, distraction techniques (engaging in enjoyable activities), and pacing strategies (gradually increasing activity levels to avoid overexertion).

- **Gradually Increasing Activity Levels:** Fear of movement is a common response to chronic pain, but avoiding activity can actually worsen pain and disability over time. CBT helps you gradually increase your activity levels at a pace that feels safe and manageable, ultimately helping you overcome fear, improve function, and regain confidence in your body.

The Benefits of CBT: Unlocking a Path to Lasting Relief

Research has consistently shown that CBT is an effective treatment for chronic pain, offering numerous benefits:

- **Reduced Pain Intensity:** CBT can help reduce the perceived intensity of pain, making it more manageable and less disruptive to your life.
- **Improved Mood and Sleep:** By addressing the emotional distress associated with pain and teaching you effective coping strategies, CBT can improve mood, reduce anxiety, and promote better sleep quality.
- **Increased Function and Activity Levels:** CBT helps you overcome fear of movement, gradually increase your activity levels, and regain

confidence in your body's ability to move and function.

- **Enhanced Sense of Control:** Perhaps most importantly, CBT empowers you with a sense of control over your pain, rather than feeling like you're at its mercy.

You don't have to navigate the challenges of chronic pain alone. Seeking guidance from a qualified therapist who specializes in CBT for pain management can equip you with the tools and strategies you need to rewire your pain response, reclaim your well-being, and create a life filled with greater ease, joy, and possibility.

Mindfulness: Finding Peace in the Midst of Pain

Our brains often spiral, obsessed with the past or the future, which can make experiencing discomfort much more intense. Mindfulness helps us break free from this constant mental loop, allowing us to reconnect with the present moment.

This practice encourages non-judgmental awareness of our thoughts, feelings, and bodily sensations. It's about observing these experiences without becoming swept away by them, allowing for greater clarity and acceptance of the present.

Consider a still lake. Its still surface allows us to see its depths. The choppy surface, on the other hand, obscures the view. Mindfulness helps to still the waves within, offering us a clearer understanding of our inner landscape.

How Mindfulness Helps with Pain Management

Mindfulness doesn't erase pain, but it can profoundly change how we relate to it, reducing its grip on our thoughts, emotions, and overall well-being.

Here's how:

- **Reducing Catastrophizing:** When we're in pain, it's easy to get caught in a cycle of negative thoughts – "This pain will never end," "I'm going to be disabled," "My life is ruined." Mindfulness helps us step back from these catastrophic thoughts, observing them without judgment and recognizing that they are simply thoughts, not facts.
- **Shifting Focus:** Pain often demands our attention, dominating our thoughts and dictating our actions. Mindfulness helps us gently shift our focus away from the pain sensations and towards other experiences – the feeling of the sun on our skin, the sound of birds singing, the taste of a delicious meal. This shift in attention doesn't negate the pain, but it helps us create a sense of space around it, reducing its power to consume us.
- **Cultivating Acceptance:** Resisting pain often

intensifies our suffering. Mindfulness helps us cultivate a sense of acceptance – not resignation, but a willingness to acknowledge the pain without judgment or resistance. This acceptance can, paradoxically, reduce the emotional distress associated with pain and make it feel more manageable.

Simple Mindfulness Practices to Try:

- **Body Scan Meditation:** This practice involves bringing your attention systematically through your body, noticing any sensations without judgment. Start at your toes and slowly move your attention upward, observing any tingling, warmth, pressure, or tension.
- **Mindful Breathing:** This simple yet powerful practice involves focusing your attention on the sensation of your breath as it enters and leaves your body. Notice the rise and fall of your chest or abdomen, the coolness of the air as you inhale, and the warmth as you exhale.
- **Mindful Walking:** This practice involves bringing your attention to the sensations of walking – the feeling of your feet on the ground, the movement of your legs, the rhythm of your breath. Notice the sights, sounds, and smells around you as you walk, engaging all your senses in the present moment.

Even a few minutes of mindful practice each day can make a profound difference in your relationship with pain, helping you cultivate a sense of peace, presence, and acceptance in the midst of discomfort.

Finding Strength in Shared Experiences: The Power of Connection

Imagine chronic pain as a heavy fog, engulfing your life in a cold, gray blanket. It can be isolating, making you feel unseen, unheard, and trapped within its silent grip. But just like sunlight cuts through fog, connection and community can illuminate your path. Sharing your struggles with others who understand the limitations, the frustrations, and the emotional toll, can offer a sense of release and validation. Support groups and online communities can provide that much-needed warmth, reminding you that you are not alone in your journey.

Support Groups: Finding Strength in Numbers

Support groups provide a unique opportunity to connect with individuals who truly "get it" – who understand the daily struggles, the emotional rollercoaster, and the often-invisible challenges of living with chronic pain.

Here are some key benefits of participating in support groups:

- **Connecting with Others Who Understand:** In a

support group, you're surrounded by people who have walked a similar path, who can empathize with your struggles, and who offer validation and encouragement.

- **Sharing Coping Strategies:** Support groups provide a platform for sharing practical tips, coping strategies, and resources for managing pain. You might learn about new therapies, relaxation techniques, or lifestyle modifications that have helped others.

- **Learning From Each Other's Experiences:** Each person's journey with pain is unique, but by sharing their stories, group members can learn from each other's successes, challenges, and insights.

- **Feeling Less Alone:** One of the most powerful benefits of support groups is the realization that you're not alone in your struggle. Sharing your experiences and hearing others' stories can reduce feelings of isolation and create a sense of connection and belonging.

- **Reducing Stigma:** Chronic pain is often misunderstood and stigmatized. Support groups can help reduce this stigma by creating a space for open and honest conversations about the realities of living with pain.

Finding Support: Connecting with Others on Your Journey

Here are some resources for finding support groups and online communities:

- **The American Chronic Pain Association (ACPA):** https://theacpa.org/ The ACPA offers a directory of support groups, as well as online resources and educational materials.
- **Pain Connection:** https://painconnection.org/ Pain Connection provides online support groups, webinars, and educational programs.
- **Facebook Groups:** Search for Facebook groups related to your specific pain condition or for general chronic pain support groups.

You don't have to navigate the challenges of chronic pain alone. Connecting with others can provide a lifeline of support, hope, and practical strategies to help you reclaim your well-being and live a more fulfilling life.

Healing from Within: Embracing a Holistic Approach to Pain Relief

The RESTORE Framework is founded on the principle that true healing encompasses the whole person – body, mind, and spirit. We recognize that chronic pain is rarely just a physical problem; it's a complex interplay of physical sensations, emotions, thoughts, beliefs, and lifestyle factors.

This holistic perspective guides everything we do at Rodrock Chiropractic. We believe that lasting relief from pain requires a multi-faceted approach that addresses not just the symptoms, but also the underlying causes, the emotional impact, and the lifestyle factors that contribute to your pain.

A Symphony of Healing: The Power of Integrating Mind and Body

Imagine trying to play a beautiful symphony with only half the orchestra. The music would be incomplete, lacking harmony and depth. Similarly, attempting to heal from chronic pain by focusing solely on the physical aspects is like playing a symphony with only half the instruments.

True healing requires the full orchestra – addressing the physical, emotional, and lifestyle factors that contribute to your pain. It's about:

- **Seeking Professional Guidance:** Connect with qualified healthcare providers, such as chiropractors, physical therapists, massage therapists, and mental health professionals, who understand the complex nature of pain and can provide personalized guidance and support.

- **Embracing a Multi-Faceted Approach:** Explore a variety of treatment modalities, including chiropractic adjustments, massage therapy, acupuncture, exercise, nutrition, stress management techniques, and mindfulness practices.
- **Cultivating Self-Compassion:** Be kind to yourself on this journey. Healing takes time, and setbacks are a normal part of the process. Celebrate your progress, acknowledge your challenges, and treat yourself with the same compassion you would offer a loved one.

Your Journey to Wholeness Starts Now

You don't have to navigate the challenges of chronic pain alone. At Rodrock Chiropractic, we offer a supportive and compassionate environment where you can explore a holistic approach to pain relief. We're here to help you address the physical, emotional, and lifestyle factors that contribute to your discomfort and empower you to reclaim your health and well-being.

We encourage you to reach out to us or connect with a qualified mental health professional to begin your journey toward wholeness today. Remember, lasting relief is possible, and you deserve to live a life free from the limitations of pain.

Amber's Testimonial: Rodrock Chiropractic's

Welcoming Office & Outstanding Care Exceeded Expectations

The entire Rodrock team is exceptional! The chiropractic and massage care I've received has been outstanding. The office is welcoming and extremely well-managed, making everything from scheduling appointments to insurance and billing details a breeze. After a significant injury, they were able to see me immediately. Thanks to their expert care, I'm back on my feet, literally! Every member of the team is kind and truly cares about me, my health, and my well-being. I highly recommend Rodrock Chiropractic!

Move with ease, live with joy. Call 785-465-5605 and let's start your journey to a pain-free life.

** Individual outcomes may differ.*

** Individual results may vary. Please review the disclaimer after the Table of Contents.*

11

EMBRACING YOUR NEW LIFE

Stepping Into a Future Free from Pain's Grip

Chronic pain can feel like a cage, keeping you trapped and holding you back. But you're not meant to live a life of limitations. There is a path forward, a chance to break free from the prison of pain. This chapter will guide you through that process – showing you how to manage the pain, build your strength, and embrace the freedom of living a life you truly want to live. We'll explore ways to reclaim your joy, rekindle your spirit, and rediscover the beauty of movement and purpose.

Shedding the Pain Identity: Releasing the Grip of the Past

Chronic pain is like a stubborn shadow, always looming, always influencing how we see ourselves and our place in the world. It can morph into a defining label, whispering, "This is who you are now." But those whispers are a lie. Pain might hold a grip on our daily lives, dictating our choices and filling our days with doctor visits and endless searches for relief. It might make us feel like we're on a treadmill of frustration, anger, and even a heavy, heart-aching sadness. But amidst this, remember, the pain does not define you. You are capable of much more than the discomfort, the limitations, and the whispers suggest. You hold within you a reservoir of strength and resilience waiting to be unleashed.

Shedding the pain identity is a process of reclaiming your true self – the person you were before pain took hold, the person you still are beneath the layers of discomfort and limitation. It's about:

- **Acknowledging the Impact:** Recognizing how pain has shaped your life, your choices, and your self-perception.
- **Releasing the Emotional Baggage:** Allowing yourself to grieve the life you thought you'd have, the experiences you missed, and the dreams you put on hold.
- **Shifting Your Perspective:** Moving from "someone living with pain" to "someone reclaiming their life."
- **Embracing a New Identity:** Rediscovering your passions, exploring new possibilities, and defining

yourself by your strengths, your values, and your dreams, not by your pain.

This process takes time, courage, and self-compassion. It's a journey of letting go of the past and embracing the potential for a new, more fulfilling future.

Rediscovering Joy: Awakening to a World of Possibilities

Pain can be a heavy chain, holding you captive in its grasp. But as its hold weakens, you feel the chains start to loosen. It's like waking up from a long, oppressive dream. Laughter bubbles up naturally, a spontaneous response to a simple, beautiful moment. You feel a renewed sense of energy, a thirst for experiences that pain had stifled. Suddenly, the world seems vibrant, alive with possibilities. You're free to embrace those things that bring you joy, to explore uncharted paths, to rediscover yourself.

Reclaiming Your Passions:

Remember those hobbies you loved, the activities that lit you up, the things you were passionate about before pain took hold? It's time to dust them off and rekindle the flame. Whether it's painting, gardening, dancing, playing music, or hiking in nature, re-engaging with your passions can reignite your sense of purpose, reconnect you with your true self, and fill your life with joy and meaning.

Exploring New Horizons:

Imagine a weight lifting from your shoulders, a newfound lightness that opens doors to unexplored landscapes. It's the feeling of freedom from the grip of pain, a sense of liberation that fuels the pursuit of your dreams. Maybe there's a dormant passion waiting to be rekindled – a musical instrument collecting dust in the attic, a dusty recipe book longing to be brought to life, or the whispering call of far-off destinations. This is your chance to say "yes" to those longings, to break free from routine, and embark on a journey of self-discovery.

Finding Joy in the Everyday:

Joy isn't just found in grand adventures or extraordinary achievements; it's also woven into the fabric of everyday life. Simple pleasures – a walk in nature, a shared meal with loved ones, a moment of laughter, a good night's sleep – can fill your days with a sense of contentment and well-being.

Here are a few ways to cultivate joy in your life:

- **Connect with Nature:** Spend time outdoors, immersing yourself in the beauty of the natural world.
- **Engage in Creative Pursuits:** Explore artistic expression through painting, writing, music, or crafts.

- **Give Back to Others:** Volunteering your time and skills can bring a sense of purpose and fulfillment.
- **Prioritize Connection:** Spend quality time with loved ones, nurture your relationships, and create shared experiences.
- **Practice Gratitude:** Take time each day to appreciate the good things in your life, no matter how small.

Rediscovering joy is an ongoing process, a journey of exploration and self-discovery. Be open to new experiences, embrace the simple pleasures, and allow yourself to be surprised by the abundance of joy that awaits you.

Reclaiming Your Body: Moving with Freedom and Joy

As pain releases its grip, you'll likely experience a profound shift, not just emotionally but also physically. Your body, no longer burdened by constant discomfort, begins to awaken, rediscovering its innate capacity for movement, strength, and vitality.

This rediscovery often starts with subtle but significant changes:

- **Increased Energy:** The energy that was once consumed by pain and inflammation becomes available for other activities, leaving you feeling more vibrant and alive.

- **Improved Mobility:** Movement becomes easier, more fluid, and more enjoyable. Stiffness and limitations gradually fade, replaced by a sense of freedom and expanded possibilities.
- **Better Sleep:** Restful sleep, once disrupted by pain, becomes more attainable, allowing your body to repair, recharge, and wake up feeling refreshed and energized.

Moving with Intention: Exploring New Ways to Connect with Your Body

You are uniquely designed, and so is the way your body wants to move. Take this newfound freedom to honor those individual needs. Pay attention to your body's whispers; a gentle stretch, a burst of energy, a craving for calm - these are its personal requests. The journey to physical well-being is paved with conscious movement. Listen, explore, and embrace your own path, one joyful step at a time.

Here are a few ideas to inspire you:

- **Dance:** Let your body move freely to the rhythm of music, expressing yourself through movement and rediscovering the joy of uninhibited expression.
- **Yoga:** This ancient practice combines physical postures, breathing exercises, and meditation,

promoting flexibility, strength, balance, and a deep connection between mind and body.

- **Hiking:** Immerse yourself in nature, enjoying the fresh air, the beauty of the trails, and the invigorating challenge of climbing hills and exploring new paths.
- **Swimming:** This low-impact activity provides a full-body workout while supporting your joints and offering a sense of weightlessness and freedom.

As you explore new ways of moving, remember to:

- **Start Slowly:** Ease into new activities gradually, honoring your body's limits and allowing time for adaptation.
- **Listen to Your Body:** Pay attention to how your body feels during and after exercise. Adjust your intensity, duration, or type of activity as needed.
- **Find Joy in the Movement:** Choose activities that you genuinely enjoy – this will make it more likely that you'll stick with them.
- **Celebrate Your Progress:** Acknowledge how far you've come and celebrate your body's strength, resilience, and adaptability.

This journey of reclaiming your body is about more than just physical fitness; it's about rediscovering the joy of movement, cultivating a deeper connection with your physical self, and celebrating the extraordinary vessel that carries you through life.

Reconnecting and Rebuilding: Strengthening Relationships After Pain

Chronic pain doesn't just affect the individual; it ripples outward, impacting relationships with loved ones, creating strain, and often leaving both parties feeling frustrated, helpless, and disconnected.

It's essential to acknowledge that pain can take a toll on relationships in many ways:

- **Irritability and Mood Changes:** Constant pain can lead to irritability, mood swings, and difficulty regulating emotions, making it challenging to engage in positive interactions with loved ones.
- **Limitations in Shared Activities:** Pain might prevent you from participating in activities you once enjoyed together, leading to feelings of isolation, resentment, and a sense of loss for both parties.
- **Emotional Burden on Caregivers:** Loved ones often take on the role of caregivers, providing physical and emotional support, which can be both rewarding and incredibly draining. This can lead

to caregiver burnout, resentment, and strain on the relationship.

Building Bridges: Pain Relief as a Catalyst for Deeper Connection

As pain recedes and you begin to reclaim your life, you'll likely find that your relationships also begin to heal and deepen.

Here's how pain relief can transform your relationships:

- **Increased Patience and Emotional Regulation:** With reduced pain, you might find that you're less irritable, more patient, and better able to regulate your emotions, allowing for more positive interactions with loved ones.
- **Renewed Energy for Shared Activities:** As your energy levels increase and your mobility improves, you can re-engage in activities you once enjoyed together, creating shared experiences, laughter, and memories.
- **Reduced Burden on Caregivers:** As you become more independent and require less assistance, your loved ones can step back from the caregiver role, reducing their burden and allowing for a more balanced and reciprocal relationship.
- **Deeper Empathy and Understanding:** Having gone through the challenges of chronic pain, you

might find that you have a greater capacity for empathy and understanding, not just for your own experiences but also for the struggles of others.

Communicating with Love: Nurturing Your Connections

Open and honest communication is crucial for rebuilding and strengthening relationships after pain.

Here are a few tips:

- **Share Your Experiences:** Talk to your loved ones about your pain journey – the challenges you've faced, the emotions you've experienced, and the ways in which pain has impacted your life and your relationships.
- **Acknowledge Their Perspectives:** Listen to your loved ones' perspectives and validate their experiences. They might have also felt frustrated, helpless, or burdened during your pain journey.
- **Express Gratitude:** Let your loved ones know how much you appreciate their support, their patience, and their understanding.
- **Seek Professional Guidance:** If you're struggling to communicate effectively or if your relationships are strained, consider seeking guidance from a therapist or counselor who specializes in couples or family therapy.

Healing is not just an individual journey; it's a shared experience that can bring you closer to your loved ones and create a deeper, more meaningful connection.

Building a Brighter Future: Embracing Limitless Possibilities

The darkness of chronic pain may finally be fading, replaced by the shimmering promise of a new beginning. It's a chance to reclaim your life, free from the constraints that pain imposed. Imagine: new goals beckoning, ambitions reignited, a life that truly embodies the person you are meant to be. No longer shackled by pain's grip, your vision broadens, embracing the countless possibilities that await.

Dreaming Big: Setting New Goals

What have you always longed to do, but pain held you back? Perhaps it's traveling to a far-off destination, pursuing a new career path, rekindling a neglected passion, or simply spending more quality time with loved ones. Whatever your aspirations, now is the time to embrace them, to set new goals, and to take those first steps towards making them a reality.

Your goals don't have to be grand or ambitious; they can be simple, everyday aspirations—spending more time in nature, learning a new skill, reading that book you've been meaning to pick up, or simply savoring each moment with greater presence and gratitude.

Maintaining Momentum: The Importance of Ongoing Care

Remember, healing is a journey, not a destination. Even as pain subsides, it's crucial to continue nourishing your body, mind, and spirit to maintain your progress and prevent setbacks.

Here are some key principles to remember:

- **Continue Healthy Habits:** Keep nourishing your body with a healthy diet, engaging in regular exercise, prioritizing sleep, and managing stress.
- **Stay Connected with Your Support System:** Maintain relationships with healthcare providers who support your holistic well-being, and lean on loved ones for encouragement and understanding.
- **Seek Support When Needed:** Don't hesitate to reach out for help if you encounter challenges or setbacks.
- **Embrace a Lifestyle of Wellness:** View health as an ongoing practice, a lifelong commitment to making choices that support your overall well-being.

Embracing a Life of Limitless Potential

Chronic pain doesn't have to define you. It might have been a challenging chapter in your story, but it doesn't have to dictate the entire narrative. By embracing the RESTORE Framework – a holistic approach that empowers you to heal from within – you can create a future filled with joy, vitality, and limitless potential.

This is your time to shine, to embrace the possibilities, and to live a life that reflects your true self – a life full of purpose, passion, and the freedom to move, explore, and experience the world with an open heart.

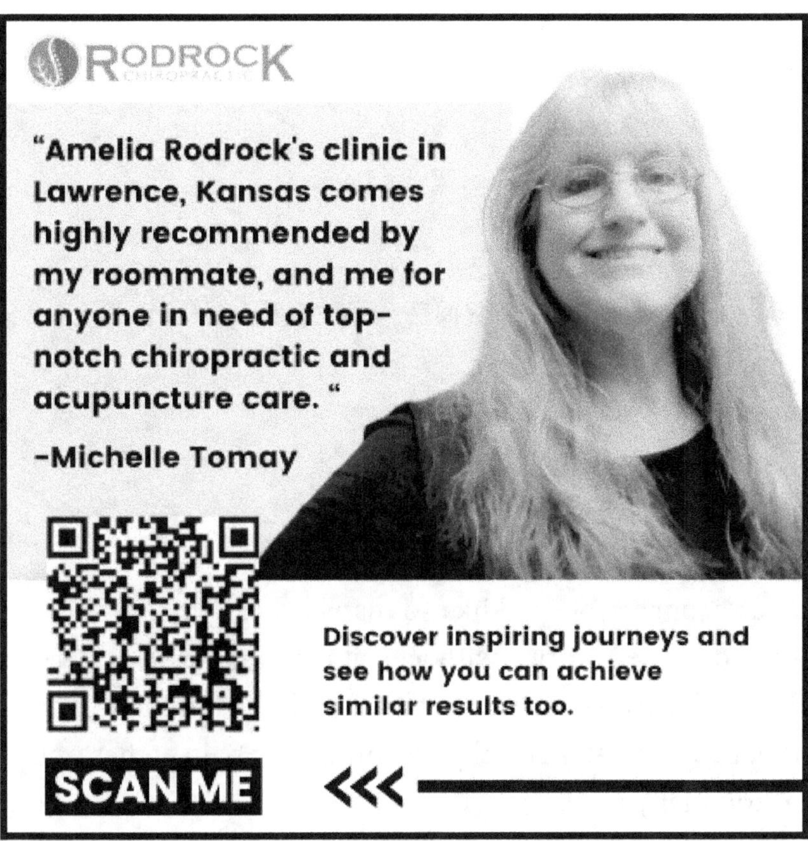

Say goodbye to discomfort, hello to vitality. Call 785-465-5605 and discover lasting relief.

** Individual results may vary. Please review the disclaimer after the Table of Contents.*

12

YOUR JOURNEY STARTS NOW

Sarah's journey started like so many others we see. She walked into our office with a hesitant gait, her shoulders slumped forward, her face etched with the familiar blend of pain and frustration that chronic back pain etches onto far too many lives.

Years of battling debilitating lower back pain had taken their toll. Simple activities like playing with her children or enjoying a walk in the park had become distant memories, replaced by a constant cycle of doctor visits, medications, and fleeting moments of relief.

"I'm ready to give up," she confessed, her voice laced with despair. "I don't think anything can help me."

But as we listened to her story, as we saw the flicker of hope beneath the surface of her resignation, we knew that Sarah wasn't ready to give up. She was ready for a different approach, a path that addressed not just her symptoms but also the underlying causes of her pain, a journey that empowered her to reclaim her health and her life.

And that's precisely what the RESTORE Framework offered. Over the next several months, we witnessed a remarkable transformation. As Sarah diligently followed the program, embracing gentle exercises, mindful movement, and nourishing food choices, the pain that had once controlled her life began to recede. Her posture improved, her energy levels soared, and the joy that had been dimmed by years of discomfort began to shine through once more.

One day, Sarah walked into our office with a radiant smile and a spring in her step. "I can't believe how much better I feel!" she exclaimed. "I'm finally living my life again!" While individual results can vary, Sarah's story is a testament to the transformative power of making a commitment to your well-being, of embarking on a journey of healing and embracing the possibilities that await on the other side of pain.

Embracing the Path: Your First Steps Towards Lasting Relief

You've read about the challenges of chronic pain, explored the limitations of quick fixes, and discovered the power of the RESTORE Framework. Now, it's time to take the first step on *your* journey toward lasting relief and a life free from pain's grip.

Making the Commitment: A Decision for a Better Future

Living with chronic pain isn't about wishing it away. It's about making a powerful choice – to prioritize your well-being. It's not a straight line to a pain-free life; it's a winding path filled with twists and turns. But each step you take, every small decision to move your body gently, nourish your spirit, and seek support, is a step toward healing. Remember, your body has an incredible ability to heal, and your commitment to its journey is the most powerful tool you have.

This commitment involves:

- **Acknowledging the Need for Change:** Recognizing that your current approach might not be serving you and that you're ready to explore a new path.
- **Setting Realistic Expectations:** Understanding that healing takes time, effort, and patience. There will be ups and downs, setbacks, and plateaus along the way.
- **Investing in Your Well-being:** This might involve prioritizing healthy habits, seeking professional guidance, making time for self-care, or exploring new therapies and modalities.

Embracing the Process: Finding Joy in the Journey

Think of healing as a puzzle. It might take time, effort, and a few missteps to assemble all the pieces. You might feel discouraged along the way, but each attempt, every bit of progress, is a victory. Embrace the journey, with all its twists and turns. Celebrate each small success, learn from the stumbles, and know that the true beauty lies not in reaching the finish line, but in the process itself.

Here's how to shift your perspective:

- **Focus on Progress, Not Perfection:** Acknowledge and celebrate every step forward, no matter how small.
- **Practice Self-Compassion:** Be kind to yourself, especially during challenging times. Remember that healing is a process, not an event, and setbacks are a normal part of the journey.
- **Find Joy in the Small Things:** Notice the moments of ease, the glimpses of progress, and the subtle shifts in your well-being. These small joys can fuel your motivation and keep you moving forward.

Setting Achievable Milestones: Breaking Down Your Goals

Overwhelm is a common obstacle on the path to healing. Looking at the big picture – eliminating all pain, achieving perfect health, transforming your life – can feel daunting and insurmountable.

Breaking down your goals into smaller, achievable milestones can make the journey feel more manageable, boost your confidence, and create a sense of momentum as you progress.

Consider setting SMART goals:

- **Specific:** Clearly define what you want to achieve.
- **Measurable:** Make your goals quantifiable so you can track your progress.
- **Achievable:** Set goals that are challenging but realistic within your current abilities and resources.
- **Relevant:** Ensure your goals align with your values, priorities, and overall vision for your health.
- **Time-Bound:** Set a realistic timeframe for achieving your goals.

The Importance of Patience: Allowing Time for Healing

In our fast-paced world, we're conditioned to expect instant gratification. But healing, especially from chronic pain, is a process that unfolds over time. It's like planting a seed – you can't force a flower to bloom overnight. It needs nurturing, patience, and time to grow.

Cultivating patience on your healing journey involves:

- **Trusting the Process:** Have faith that your body is capable of healing and that the steps you're taking are moving you in the right direction, even if you don't see immediate results.
- **Shifting Your Perspective:** View setbacks as opportunities for learning and growth, not as failures.
- **Celebrating Small Victories:** Acknowledge and appreciate every step forward, no matter how small.

Remember, your journey is unique. There's no set timeline for healing. Be patient with yourself, be persistent in your efforts, and celebrate every milestone along the way.

Implementing the RESTORE Framework: A Roadmap to Lasting Relief

You've learned about the principles of the RESTORE Framework – a holistic approach that addresses the physical, emotional, and lifestyle factors that contribute to pain. Now, it's time to put those principles into action, integrating them into your daily life and embarking on a journey toward lasting relief and optimal well-being.

Practical Tips for Everyday Living: Making RESTORE a Way of Life

The RESTORE Framework isn't just a set of treatments; it's a philosophy, a way of approaching life that prioritizes your health and empowers you to make choices that support your body's natural healing abilities. Here are some practical tips to integrate RESTORE principles into your daily routine:

- **Move with Intention:** Incorporate regular movement into your day, even if it's just a few minutes of stretching, walking, or gentle exercise.
- **Nourish Your Body:** Choose whole, unprocessed foods that provide the nutrients your spine and joints need to thrive. Limit inflammatory foods like processed snacks, sugary drinks, and unhealthy fats.
- **Prioritize Rest and Recovery:** Ensure you're getting adequate sleep, allowing your body time to repair and recharge. Incorporate relaxation techniques into your day to manage stress and calm your nervous system.
- **Create an Ergonomic Environment:** Assess your workspace and home environment, making adjustments to support your posture and minimize strain on your body.
- **Tune into Your Body's Signals:** Pay attention to how your body feels. Notice any pain, stiffness, or

limitations, and address them promptly. Don't ignore your body's whispers; they often hold valuable insights into your needs.

- **Seek Professional Guidance:** Don't hesitate to reach out to your healthcare team for support, adjustments, or guidance as needed.

Tracking Your Progress: Celebrating the Small Wins

As you implement the RESTORE Framework, it's essential to track your progress, not just to monitor your pain levels but also to acknowledge and celebrate your accomplishments. This can help you stay motivated, identify what's working, and make adjustments along the way.

Here are a few ways to track your progress:

- **Pain Journal:** Keep a journal to record your pain levels, activities that trigger pain, treatments you've tried, and any other relevant observations about your well-being.
- **Pain Scale:** Use a numerical pain scale (0-10) to rate your pain intensity at various times throughout the day.
- **Activity Tracking:** Note how your ability to participate in activities you enjoy has changed over time. Are you able to walk further, stand longer, or engage in activities you previously avoided?

- **Mood and Sleep Tracking:** Monitor your mood, energy levels, and sleep quality. These factors are often intertwined with pain and can provide valuable insights into your overall progress.

Adjusting As You Go: Honoring Your Body's Feedback

There will be ups and downs, plateaus, and unexpected challenges along the way. The RESTORE Framework isn't about rigidly adhering to a set plan; it's about listening to your body's feedback, making adjustments as needed, and finding what works best for you.

Don't be afraid to:

- **Modify Your Approach:** If a particular exercise, therapy, or lifestyle change isn't working for you, explore alternatives or adjust the intensity or frequency.
- **Communicate with Your Healthcare Team:** Share your experiences, challenges, and successes with your healthcare providers. They can help you adjust your treatment plan, offer support, and guide you towards optimal outcomes.
- **Be Patient and Persistent:** Healing takes time. Don't get discouraged if you encounter setbacks or plateaus. Stay committed to your goals, celebrate your progress, and trust in your body's innate healing abilities.

Celebrating Your Successes: Acknowledging How Far You've Come

It's easy to get caught up in the daily challenges of managing pain, focusing on what still needs to be done rather than acknowledging how far you've come. Celebrating your successes, no matter how small, is essential for staying motivated, building confidence, and reinforcing positive changes.

Take time to appreciate:

- **Reduced Pain Levels:** Even a slight decrease in pain intensity can make a significant difference in your quality of life.
- **Increased Mobility:** Celebrate your ability to move more freely, participate in activities you enjoy, and reclaim your independence.
- **Improved Mood and Sleep:** Acknowledge the positive impact of reduced pain on your emotional well-being, energy levels, and sleep quality.
- **Newfound Confidence:** Recognize the strength, resilience, and determination you've demonstrated throughout your healing journey.

You are the author of your healing story. Write it with patience, perseverance, and a celebration of every step that brings you closer to a pain-free, vibrant life.

Staying on the Path: Navigating the Long-Term Journey of Healing

Healing from chronic pain is not a one-time event; it's an ongoing journey, a commitment to making choices that support your well-being and prevent pain from reclaiming its grip on your life. This path can be challenging, with inevitable ups and downs, moments of doubt, and times when you might feel tempted to revert to old habits.

Avoiding Common Pitfalls: Navigating Roadblocks on Your Path

The path to pain relief is rarely linear. It's a winding road with twists, turns, and unexpected obstacles along the way. Here are a few common pitfalls to watch out for:

- **The Quick-Fix Mentality:** Be wary of promises of instant cures or miraculous solutions. True healing takes time, effort, and a multi-faceted approach.
- **Ignoring Your Body's Signals:** It's easy to slip back into old habits of ignoring pain or pushing through discomfort. Remember, pain is a messenger, a signal that something needs attention.
- **Self-Blame and Negative Self-Talk:** Don't beat yourself up for setbacks or plateaus. Healing is a process, not a performance. Be kind to yourself, and celebrate your progress.

- **Isolation and Lack of Support:** Chronic pain can be isolating. Don't try to navigate this journey alone. Reach out to your healthcare team, loved ones, or support groups when you need encouragement, guidance, or a listening ear.

Lifelong Learning: Staying Curious About Your Health

Your body is constantly changing, adapting, and evolving. What works for you today might not work as effectively tomorrow. Embracing a mindset of lifelong learning allows you to stay informed about your health, explore new therapies and strategies, and adapt your approach as needed.

Here are a few ways to continue learning:

- **Stay Informed:** Read books, articles, and reputable websites about pain management, nutrition, exercise, and holistic health.
- **Attend Workshops or Webinars:** Many healthcare providers offer workshops or webinars on topics related to pain relief, stress management, and healthy living.
- **Explore New Modalities:** Be open to trying new therapies or techniques that might complement your existing treatment plan.
- **Ask Questions:** Don't hesitate to ask your healthcare providers questions about your

condition, treatment options, and ways to optimize your health.

Imagine a life where pain no longer holds you back, a life filled with vitality, connection, and joy. This vision can become your reality when you embrace lifelong learning, seek support from those who understand, and cultivate a community that empowers your healing journey.

A Final Word of Encouragement: Embracing the Power Within

As you close this book, we hope you're filled with a sense of hope, empowerment, and a renewed belief in your body's extraordinary capacity for healing. The journey to lasting relief from spine and joint pain might not be easy, but it's a journey worth taking – a path that leads not just to reduced discomfort but to a more vibrant, fulfilling, and joyful life.

Remember these key truths as you move forward:

- **You Are Not Alone:** Millions of people struggle with pain, and countless others have found lasting relief through holistic approaches that address the root cause, not just the symptoms.
- **Your Body is Resilient:** Your body is a remarkable self-healing organism, capable of extraordinary

repair and regeneration when given the right support.

- **You Have the Power to Choose:** Every day, you make choices that impact your health and well-being. Embrace those choices with intention, prioritize your needs, and trust in your ability to create positive change.

Ready to Take the Next Step?

Deepen Your Knowledge with Our Masterclass: If you're eager to learn more about the RESTORE Framework, our holistic approach to pain relief, and practical strategies for reclaiming your health, we invite you to sign up for our exclusive masterclass. In this in-depth session, we'll delve deeper into the principles we've discussed in this book, share valuable insights, answer your questions, and provide personalized guidance.

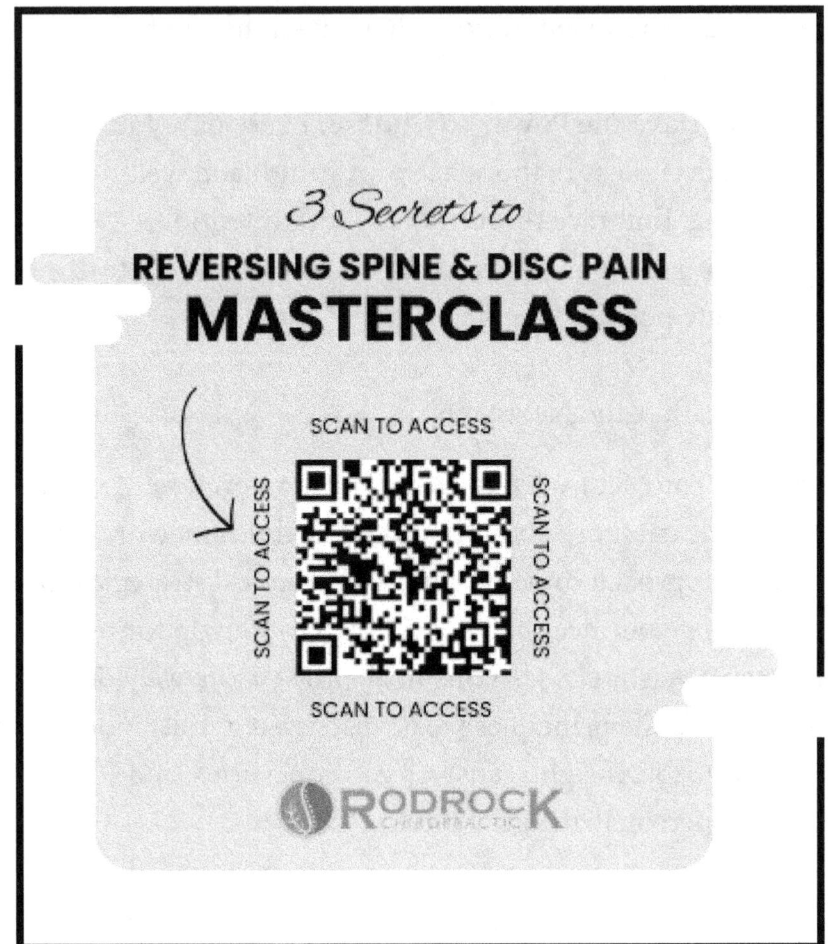

Schedule an Appointment – Let's Begin Your Journey Together: We're here to support you every step of the way on your path to lasting relief and optimal well-being. Schedule an appointment at Rodrock Chiropractic today, and let's work together to create a personalized plan that addresses your unique needs and helps you reclaim a life free from pain's limitations. Please note that while we strive to provide the best possible care, individual results may vary and are not guaranteed.

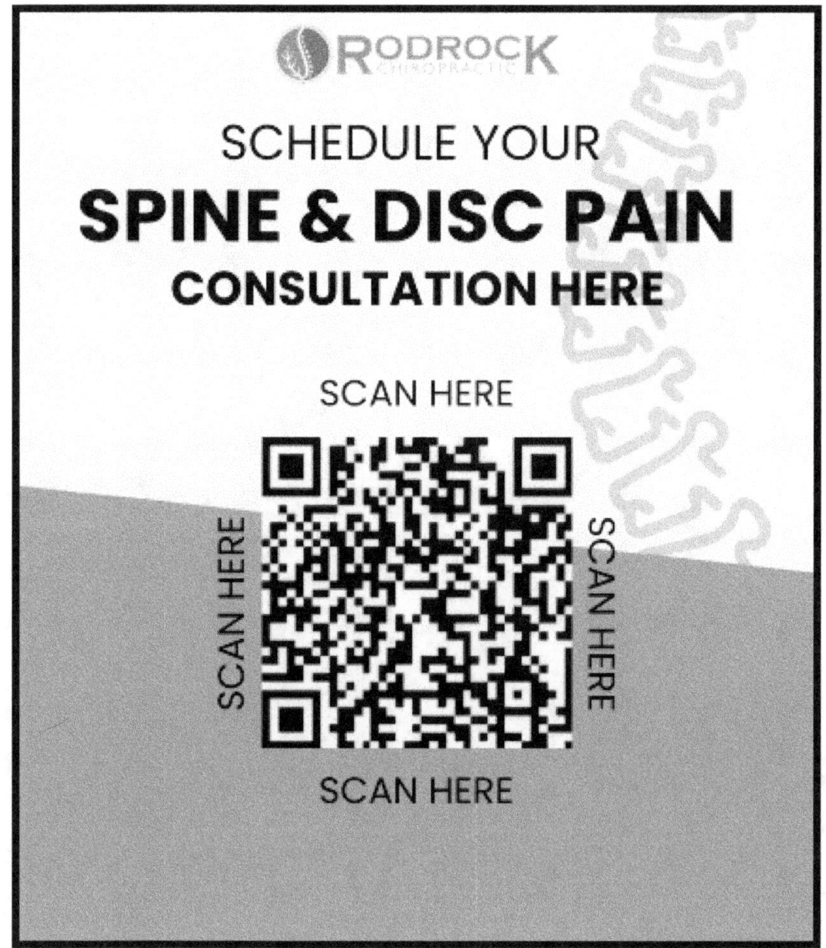

Your journey starts now! Take that first step, embrace the possibilities, and trust in the power within you to heal and thrive. We're excited to be part of your transformation!